FIRST AID
PRINCIPLES
AND
PROCEDURES

FIRST AID PRINCIPLES AND PROCEDURES

Pamela Bakhaus doCarmo
University of Maryland
Angelo T. Patterson

PRENTICE-HALL, INC.   ENGLEWOOD CLIFFS, NEW JERSEY

Library of Congress Cataloging in Publication Data

DoCarmo, Pamela B   date
   First aid principles and procedures.

   Bibliography: p. 225
   Includes index.
   1. First aid in illness and injury. I. Patterson,
Angelo T., date   joint author. II. Title.
[DNLM: 1. First aid. WA292 D636f]
RC87.D64 1975   614.8′8   75-20396
ISBN 0-13-317941-9
ISBN 0-13-317933-8 pbk.

© 1976 by PRENTICE-HALL, INC., *Englewood Cliffs, N.J.*

All rights reserved.
No part of this book may be reproduced in any form
or by any means without permission in writing
from the publisher.

10 9 8 7 6 5 4 3 2 1

Printed in the United States of America

Prentice-Hall International, Inc., *London*
Prentice-Hall of Australia, Pty. Ltd., *Sydney*
Prentice-Hall of Canada, Ltd., *Toronto*
Prentice-Hall of India Private Limited, *New Delhi*
Prentice-Hall of Japan, Inc., *Tokyo*
Prentice-Hall of Southeast Asia (Pte.), *Singapore*

CONTENTS

PREFACE ix

{ 1 }

BASIC PRINCIPLES OF FIRST AID 1

    Responsibilities at the Scene   3
    Activating the Emergency Medical System   4
    Evaluating the Injured and Ill   5
    Priorities for First Aid Care   9
    Procedures at the Scene   12
    Legal Liability   12

{ 2 }

CARDIOPULMONARY RESUSCITATION   15

    Respiratory Arrest   15
    Artificial Ventilation   19
    Café Coronary   28
    Hyperventilation   31
    Cardiac Arrest   33
    Cardiac Massage (External Heart Compression)   34
    Witnessed Cardiac Arrest   42
    Initiating and Terminating Cardiopulmonary Resuscitation   43

{ 3 }

HEMORRHAGE CONTROL   45

    Circulation of Blood   46
    Classification of Hemorrhage   46
    External Hemorrhage   46
    Amputations   53
    Nose Bleeds   53
    Internal Hemorrhage   54

{ 4 }

SOFT TISSUE INJURIES   57

    Closed Wounds   57
    Open Wounds   58
    Infection   61
    Special Wounds   63

{ 5 }

SHOCK   77

    Traumatic Shock   77
    Cardiogenic Shock   82
    Anaphylactic Shock   82
    Emotional Shock   84
    Psychogenic Shock (Fainting)   84
    Neurogenic Shock   86
    Shock Caused by Electrical Contact   86

{ 6 }

SKELETAL SYSTEM INJURIES   89

    Causes of Fractures   89
    Types of Fractures   90
    Indicators of Fractures   92
    Procedures for Closed Fractures   95
    Procedures for Open Fractures   96
    Special Fractures   96
    Injuries Related to the Skeletal System   101

{ 7 }

BURNS AND EXPOSURE 105

    Adverse Effects of Heat 105
    Heat Exhaustion 106
    Heat Stroke 107
    Heat Cramps 108
    Burns 108
    Adverse Effects of Cold 114

{ 8 }

POISONINGS 119

    Poison Control Centers 119
    Poison Entry Routes 121
    Ingested Poisons 121
    Inhaled Poisons 128
    Injected Poisons 131
    Absorbed Poisons 131

{ 9 }

MEDICAL EMERGENCIES 135

    General Unconsciousness 135
    Diabetes 141
    Convulsions 143
    Heart Attacks 145
    Cerebral Vascular Accident 148
    Appendicitis 150

{ 10 }

PSYCHOLOGICAL EMERGENCIES 151

    Emotional First Aid 151
    Alcohol Reactions 154
    Drug Reactions 157
    Suicide 157

{ 11 }

EMERGENCY CHILDBIRTH   163

    Development of the Baby   163
    The Birth Process   164
    Pre-Birth Emergencies   171
    Delivery Complications   171

{ 12 }

FIRST AID PRACTICAL SKILLS   179

    Bandaging   179
    Splinting   188
    Transporting   198

APPENDIXES   207

    A: The Skeletal System   209
    B: The Heart   210
    C: The Circulatory System   211
    D: The Respiratory System   212

GLOSSARY   213

SELECTED BIBLIOGRAPHY   225

INDEX   235

PREFACE

Although we live in an era of rapid transportation and competent medical care, there are often times when professional assistance is delayed or even unavailable. Proper immediate action by an informed layman may make the difference between whether a life is lost or saved, or whether an injury or illness is aggravated to the point of partial or total, temporary or permanent, disability. Moreover, needless pain and suffering may well be avoided, thus minimizing the physical and emotional consequences of trauma and sickness. Accidents are responsible for over 115,000 deaths annually, and millions more are being injured to some degree, the majority from actions within the home or from the motor vehicle.

Although it is impossible to estimate the number of persons who might have been saved with prompt attention, the need to train more individuals in the proper procedures at the scene of an injury or illness is evident. To substantiate this, the Department of Transportation's Highway Safety Program Standard on Driver Education encourages all students to enroll in a course in first aid. Recent legislation requires the presence of trained first aiders in all aspects of industry.

The general aim of *First Aid Principles and Procedures* is to provide a text for college students which focuses on those areas of emergency care in which they are most directly involved. The authors do not claim to present anything new or different in first aid, but rather to focus on the college student's needs and level of ability. Other first aid texts are available, but they are designed for use by specialists such as medical corpsmen, emergency medical technicians, paramedics, rescue squads, police and fire personnel, and therefore are required to be treatment and transportation orientated. Our text is designed for use in basic first aid courses which are being offered by today's colleges and universities.

The last few years have seen a tremendous advance in medical knowledge, with new life-saving techniques becoming available to the layman—perhaps the greatest of these being cardiopulmonary resuscitation. The authors firmly believe that mature young people, when properly trained, can perform these techniques effectively. Our book also focuses on the emergency procedures to be followed when there is evidence of alcohol or drug abuse. Also discussed is the nationwide emergency medical system being developed by the United States Department of Transportation. We feel certain that lay first aid is the key to the success of this program.

The latest medical concept in the treatment of trauma victims emphasizes *total care*. The injured individual, immediately upon entrance into a specialized medical facility, receives all of the medical care necessary to correct his injuries. The first aider must also try to view the trauma victim in this manner. He should examine the individual for all injuries and care for them to the best of his ability. However, in presenting the various first aid techniques and procedures, it is difficult to take this approach. For this reason the authors have retained the traditional systemic and disease categories for discussion purposes. It is up to the individual first aid instructors to correlate this material into a total picture, and we strongly recommend that they do so.

Several anatomical drawings have also been included as an aid to both instructor and student. Their use will depend upon the emphasis and focus of the first aid course. Some courses are taught on a very general anatomical and physiological level whereas other courses discuss in detail the anatomical and physiological changes occurring in trauma and disease.

The authors would like to thank Diane Lewis for her assistance in typing the manuscript and Hilda Tauber of Prentice-Hall, Inc. for her patient editing. Special thanks go to Elizabeth Warnke and Finley doCarmo for their constant encouragement during the writing and revision of the manuscript. We also wish to thank the Robert J. Brady Company, Bowie, Md. for permission to use illustrations from *Emergency Care* by Harvey Grant and Robert Murray.

FIRST AID PRINCIPLES AND PROCEDURES

{ 1 }

BASIC PRINCIPLES OF FIRST AID

With the advent of the Department of Transportation has come a closer scrutiny of the emergency medical services available to individuals who are injured or taken ill. In many parts of the country adequate services are lacking and what is available is of minimal quality. The Department of Transportation's Standard Eleven, Emergency Medical Services, attempts to establish a nationwide emergency medical service system whereby all individuals in need of medical assistance will receive prompt and efficient service from the time of recognition of need through hospital care and rehabilitation. A sophisticated system involving communication networks, ground ambulances, helicopters, specialty trauma hospitals, general hospitals, and trained personnel is emerging. Much time, effort, and money have been directed into improving the emergency medical service system, with the goal of reducing to a minimum the number of needless deaths and permanent disabilities which occur annually.

But no matter how sophisticated the system becomes, the key to its success lies with the general public. It is increasingly important that the ordinary lay person be able to recognize an emergency, that he or she* knows how the emergency system operates and is able to work with it effectively. In this light first aid training becomes essential for everyone. Although ambulances and emergency medical technicians with advanced training and equipment are becoming more available, it is still the first

---

*Throughout the rest of the book only masculine designations will be used, for grammatical simplicity.

[2] Basic Principles of First Aid

aider who must initially recognize the injury or illness and give the immediate care necessary until the system is activated and professional help arrives.

First aid is the prompt, efficient care of an individual, whether injured or ill, until medical assistance becomes available. This does not imply, however, that medical assistance, especially in the form of an ambulance or hospital, will be required in all instances. Realistically, many emergency situations that occur are relatively minor and can be handled effectively by the individual or his family. What is important for the first aider is to be able to recognize *life-threatening* illnesses and injuries, and to maintain these victims until medical assistance becomes available. Properly applied first aid techniques can restore breathing and heart beat, control hemorrhage, prevent or reduce shock, protect open wounds from contamination, minimize fracture damage, and comfort the stricken person.

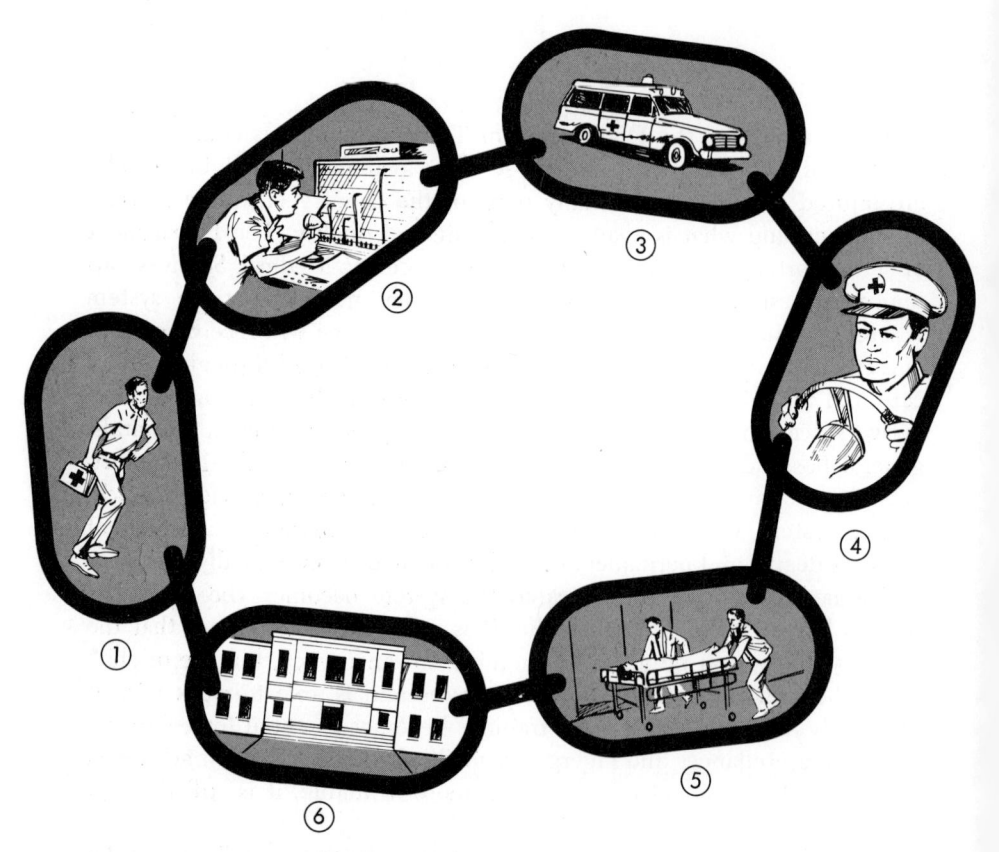

Figure 1.1 Emergency medical system.

First aid is the initial step in the general care of the injured or ill. Emergency care performed by an emergency medical technician goes a step further; it not only continues the care begun by the first aider but also packages, extricates, and transports the ill or injured to a medical facility. Definitive professional care continues where emergency care leaves off, providing assistance in the form of medication, intravenous fluids, sutures, surgery, and other medical procedures necessary to maintain and restore the individual. Figure 1.1 shows the elements in the chain of a typical emergency medical system.

RESPONSIBILITIES AT THE SCENE

When a first aider comes upon an illness or injury situation, his basic responsibilities are:

1. To protect the individual from further harm.
2. To maintain life or attempt to restore life.
3. To comfort and reassure the individual.
4. To activate the emergency medical system.

It is difficult to list in any specific order the steps to be performed at the scene of an injury or illness, because this depends upon the circumstances. In some instances relatively little can or needs to be done by the first aider to alleviate the situation; in other cases there may be almost too much for one person to handle. When the first aider comes upon an illness or injury situation, he should try first of all to find out all he can about what has happened to the victim. This may be accomplished by: (1) asking the individual, if he is conscious, what has happened and whether he hurts anywhere; (2) asking bystanders what has happened; (3) observing the individual for obvious signs of injury (for example, cyanosis or hemorrhage); and (4) evaluating the situation itself (collision, fall, poisoning, and so on). From this information the first aider can decide what assistance is necessary, that is, whether to activate the emergency medical system and whether to assist the injured or ill individual by rendering care at the scene.

Having determined that both forms of assistance are required, the first aider must next decide whether to remain at the scene and assist the injured or ill, or leave to activate the system. In most instances a bystander can be sent to activate the system while the first aider assists those who require attention. In that case the first aider must see to it that the bystander who goes to activate the system knows how to do it properly and has been given the available information necessary for proper activation.

Basic Principles of First Aid

If there is no one available for assistance, the first aider's responsibility is to stay with the injured or ill, stabilize them, then activate the system, returning to the scene as quickly as possible. It rarely occurs that there are no bystanders present, although first aiders are not always among them.

ACTIVATING THE EMERGENCY MEDICAL SYSTEM

Before activating the emergency medical system the first aider should obtain some basic facts as to: (1) what has happened; (2) how serious the injuries are, and (3) how many individuals will need assistance. It would be inadequate to activate the system without this information.

The emergency medical system is emerging throughout the United States in differing forms and at varying rates of progress. The first aider should quickly familiarize himself with how the system operates in his community or in any new locality in which he arrives. In most parts of the United States the system may be activated by telephoning a designated emergency number. This telephone number is usually well publicized, and the first aider should have it available at all times. A nationwide emergency number is being established, and when the system is completed, it will be possible to dial the number 911 anywhere within the United States to request assistance in the form of ambulances, fire apparatus, and police. In the meantime, if the first aider does not know the emergency number for the locale in which he finds himself, it is best to dial "Operator" to request assistance. The operator, in turn, will connect the first aider with the proper emergency center.

Once contact has been made with an emergency center, certain information must be communicated. In order to dispatch the proper equipment and personnel, the emergency center needs to know:

1. The exact location. This is probably the single most important piece of information necessary to properly activate the emergency medical system. Delays often occur when first aiders or bystanders give an incorrect or incomplete location.
2. The circumstances—that is, what has happened. Is it a heart attack, automobile collision, drowning, and so on.
3. The number of injured or ill individuals involved.
4. The telephone number from which the call for assistance was placed. This information is required not only to help prevent false calls, but more important, so that the center may call back for additional information. If possible the first aider should remain at this telephone for approximately fifteen minutes in case additional information is necessary.

Basic Principles of First Aid   [5]

EVALUATING THE INJURED AND ILL

Three factors that will assist the first aider in appraising an illness or injury situation are: (1) the situation itself, (2) observation and examination of the individual, and (3) the vital signs which the individual exhibits.

The Situation Itself

Often the only information available to the first aider for evaluating an emergency is the environment in which the victim is found. Frequently there are no external signs of injury, and one must suspect certain injuries or illnesses based solely upon the environment. This is particularly true if the individual is elderly, or is involved in an automobile collision, or has fallen from a height, or suddenly lost consciousness.

Observation and Examination

Often there are external, visible signs of injury, for example, deformity or hemorrhage, which immediately identify the problem for the first aider. But the obvious first-sighted injury may not always be the most severe or life-threatening one. It is important that the first aider make a systematic examination (see Figure 1.2) in order to locate all possible injuries. The survey should begin at the head and proceed systematically to the entire body. The first aider should initially check for adequate breathing

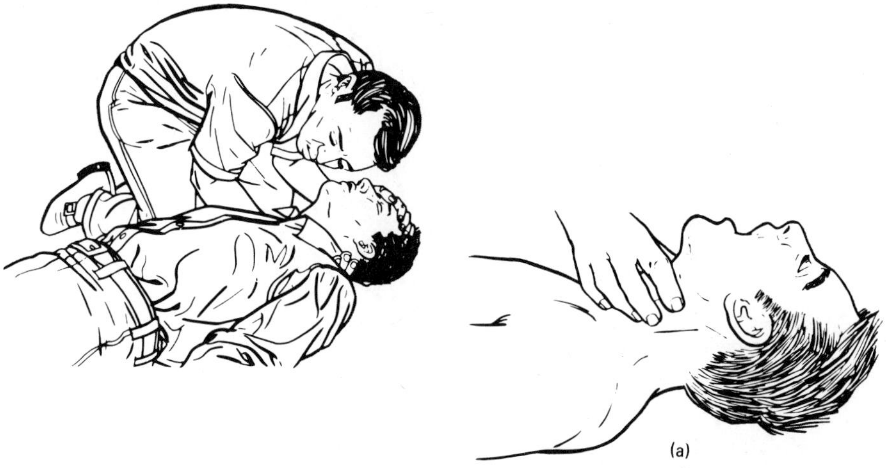

Figure 1.2 Examination of injured individual. (a) Check for breathing and pulse.

(b)

(c)

(d)

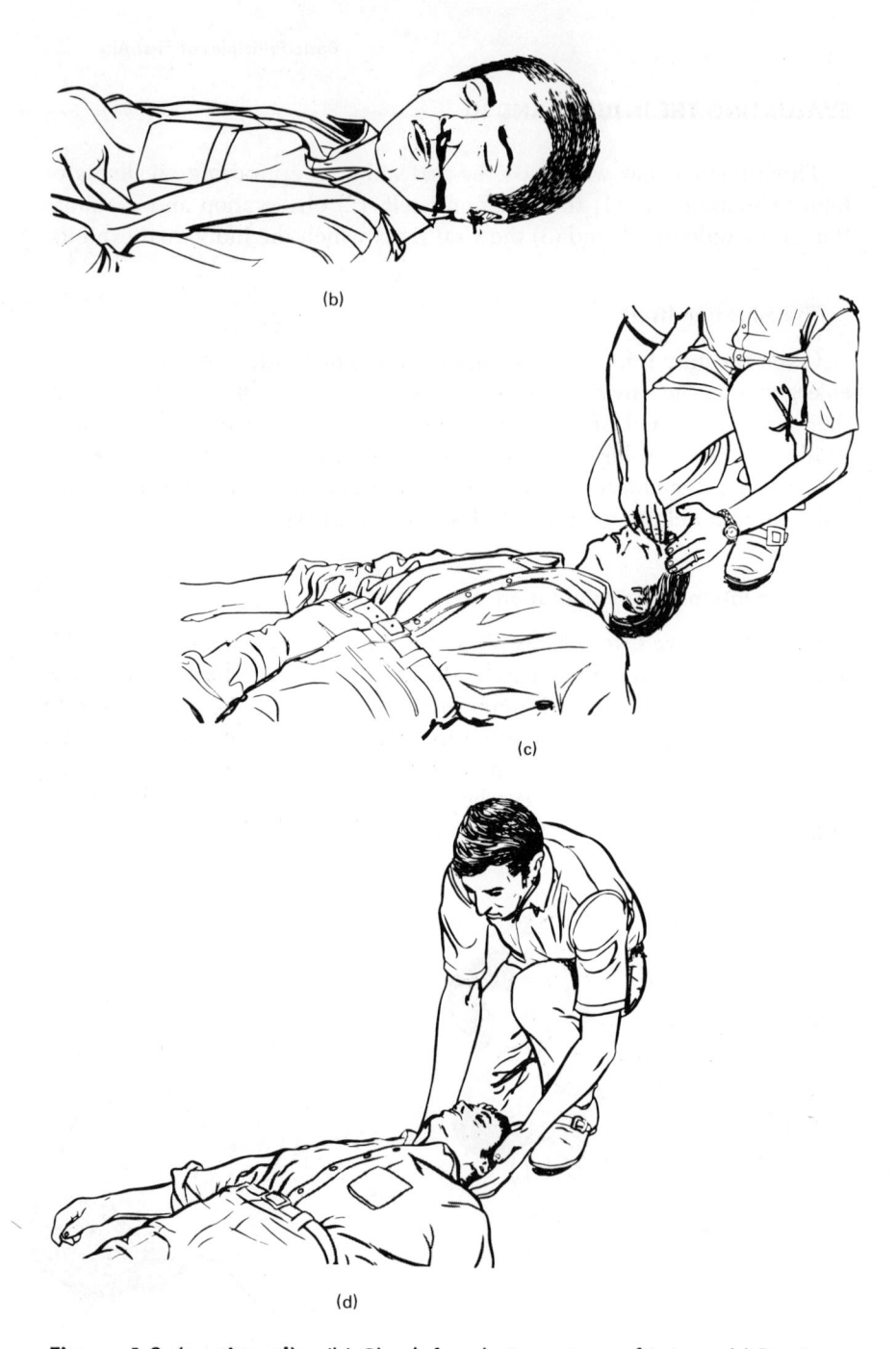

Figure 1.2 (continued) (b) Check for obvious signs of injury. (c) Begin at head examining for lacerations, contusions, swelling or depressions of body tissue. (d)-(g) Continue by examining bony surfaces of neck, chest, pelvis and extremities for depressions or protrusions. (h) Finally, check abdomen for rigidity, swelling, or spasm.

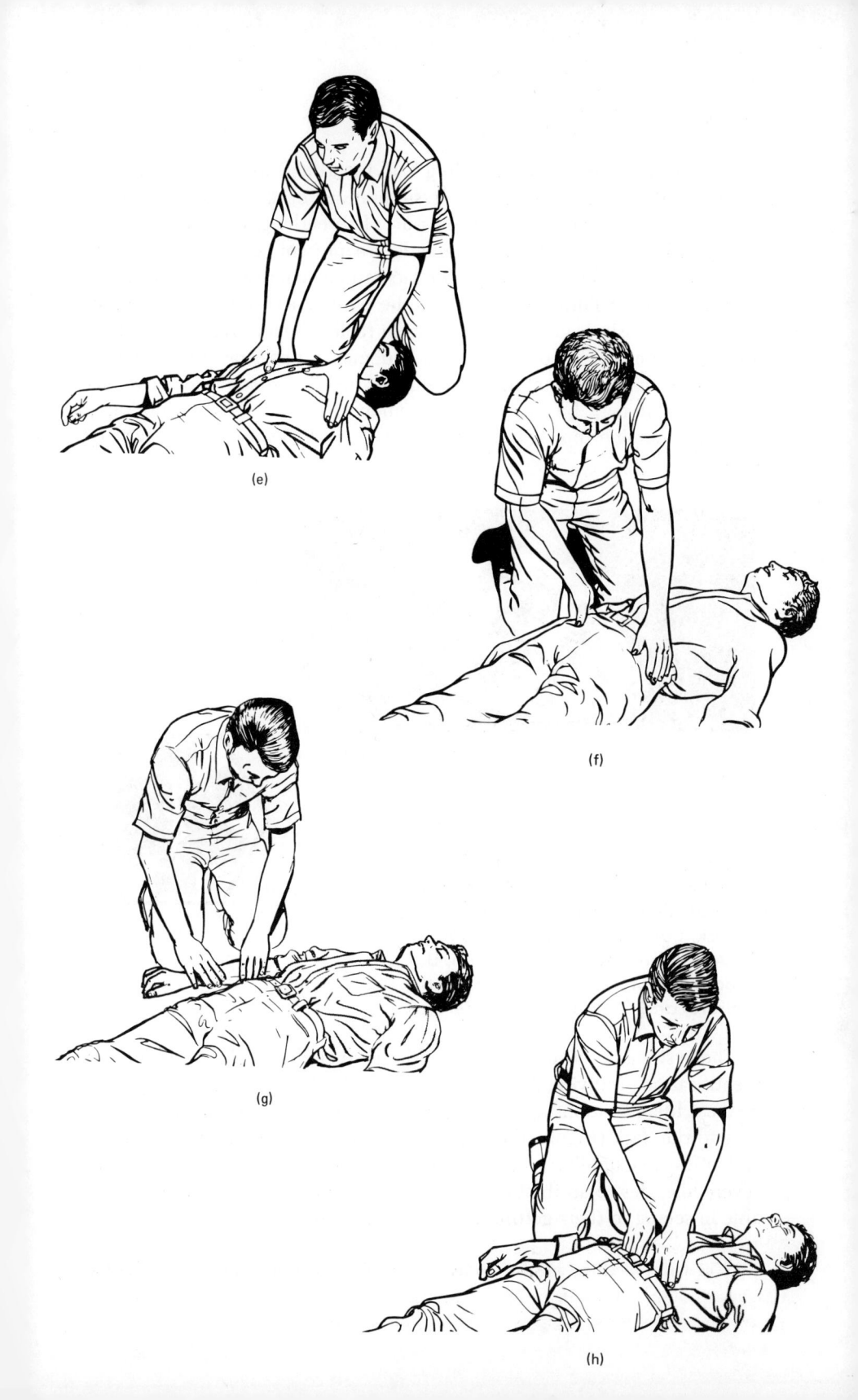

(e)

(f)

(g)

(h)

[8] Basic Principles of First Aid

and pulse and any severe bleeding.* If breathing and circulation have ceased, initiate cardiopulmonary resuscitation; or if severe bleeding is found, begin controlling it with pressure. If breathing and pulse are adequate and no severe bleeding wounds are present, continue examining the body by checking the scalp for lacerations, contusions, or depressed injuries; look for fluid escaping from the nose or ears and feel for lumps or bony protrusions in the neck, clavicle (collar bone) area, arms, pelvis, and legs. Continue by observing the abdomen for spasms and tenderness and by checking for numbness, tingling, or inability to move an extremity. Sometimes it may be necessary to remove the individual's clothing in order to examine him better. In that case try to avoid unnecessary exposure.

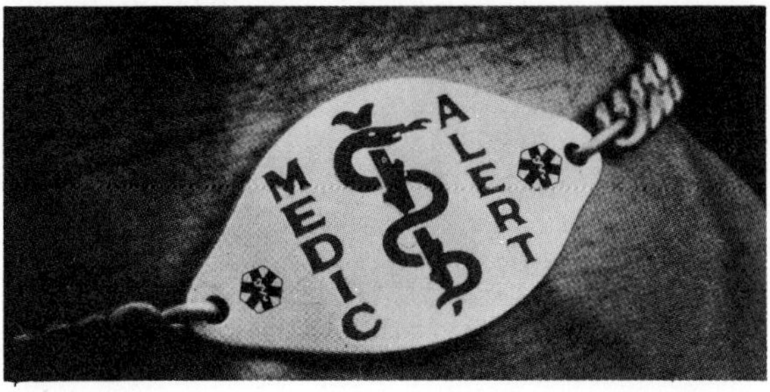

Figure 1.3 Emergency medical identification insignias. (a) Bracelet of the Medical Alert Foundation International, Turlock, California. (b) Emblem adopted by the American Medical Association, U.S. Department of Health, Education and Welfare, and the Public Health Service.

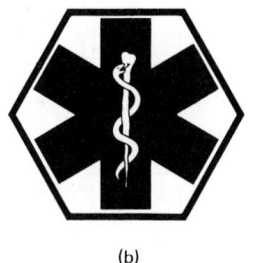

The systematic examination should also include checking for medical identification. Individuals with special medical problems often wear a medical identification tag in the form of a bracelet, or a medallion worn around the neck (Figure 1.3). Such tags identify the wearers as diabetics, epileptics, hemophiliacs, laryngectomees (neck breathers), persons with severe allergies to antibiotics, and so on. This information can be invaluable in seeing to their getting the proper care in an emergency.

*The terms *bleeding* and *hemorrhage* are used synonymously throughout the text.

Basic Principles of First Aid [9]

The Vital Signs

While the first aider is examining the individual for possible injuries, he should look, listen, and feel for certain vital body signs. Irregularities in the vital signs are indicators of changes within the body due to injury or illness. The first aider should check the following vital signs:

1. *Pulse.* If it cannot be felt at the wrist, check at the carotid artery at the neck.
2. *Respiration.* Feel for air exchange, look and listen to the rate and depth of breathing.
3. *Skin.* Observe the skin's color, temperature, and moistness.
4. *Pupils of the eye.* Observe for dilation, constriction, unequalness, and response to light.
5. *State of consciousness.* Determine whether the individual is conscious, incoherent, or unconscious.
6. *Ability to move.* Determine if the individual is able to move the arms and legs or react to external stimuli.
7. *Reaction to pain.* Ask the individual whether he feels pain or discomfort, and if so, where.

Figure 1.4 indicates some of the irregularities which may be found in the vital signs, and their possible indications for illness or injury.

Based upon the information gathered from the situation, observation and examination, and vital signs, the first aider then evaluates the seriousness or life-threatening nature of the injury or illness. A chart prepared by the American College of Surgeons (Figure 1.5) illustrates how the techniques of observation, examination, and vital signs can be used effectively. This survey is especially helpful in setting priorities in the order of care for the victims—an important consideration when the first aider is alone.

PRIORITIES FOR FIRST AID CARE

Throughout the examination and observation procedure, the first aider is attempting to locate those who are most seriously injured or ill, and to establish an order of priority for their care. *Highest priority* for receiving attention are individuals who have an obstructed airway, are having difficulty breathing, or have ceased to breathe. Closely aligned to respiratory difficulty are cardiac arrest and extremely irregular or weak heart action. Uncontrollable hemorrhage, severe head injuries, open chest or abdominal wounds, poisonings, heart attacks, and severe shock should also receive first priority. *Second priority* injuries include burns, fractures, and spinal injuries. *Lowest priority* should be assigned to minor fractures,

Figure 1.4 DIAGNOSTIC SIGNS AND THEIR SIGNIFICANCE

Diagnostic Sign	Observation	Indication
Respiration	None	Respiratory arrest
	Deep, gasping, labored	Airway obstruction; heart failure
	Bright red, frothy blood with each exhalation	Lung damage
Pulse	Absent	Cardiac arrest
	Rapid, bounding	Fright; hypertension
	Rapid, weak	Shock
Skin temperature	Hot, dry	Heat stroke; fever
	Cool, clammy	Shock
	Cold, moist	Body losing heat
	Cool, dry	Cold exposure
Skin color	Red skin	High blood pressure; carbon monoxide poisoning; heart attack; first degree burn; heat stroke
	White skin	Shock; heart attack; fright; cold exposure; heat exhaustion
	Blue skin	Asphyxia; anoxia
Pupils of the eyes	Dilated	Unconsciousness; cardiac arrest
	Constricted	Disorder affecting the central nervous system; drug use
	Unequal	Head injury; stroke
Consciousness	Brief unconsciousness	Simple fainting
	Confusion	Alcohol use; mental state; slight blow to head
	Stupor	Severe blow to head
	Deep coma	Severe brain damage; poisoning
Paralysis or loss of sensation	Lower extremities	Spinal cord injury in lower back
	Upper extremities	Spinal cord injury in neck
	Limited use of extremities	Pressure on spinal cord
	Paralysis limited to one side	Stroke; head injury with brain damage
Reaction to pain	General pain at injury sites	Injuries to the body but probably no spinal cord damage
	Local pain in extremities	Fracture; occluded artery to extremity
	No pain, but obvious sign of injury	Spinal cord damage; hysteria; violent shock; drug or alcohol abuse

Source: *Principles of First Aid: Instructor's Guide*, Robert J. Brady Company, Bowie, Md., 1973.

Figure 1.5 EXTRICATION SURVEY

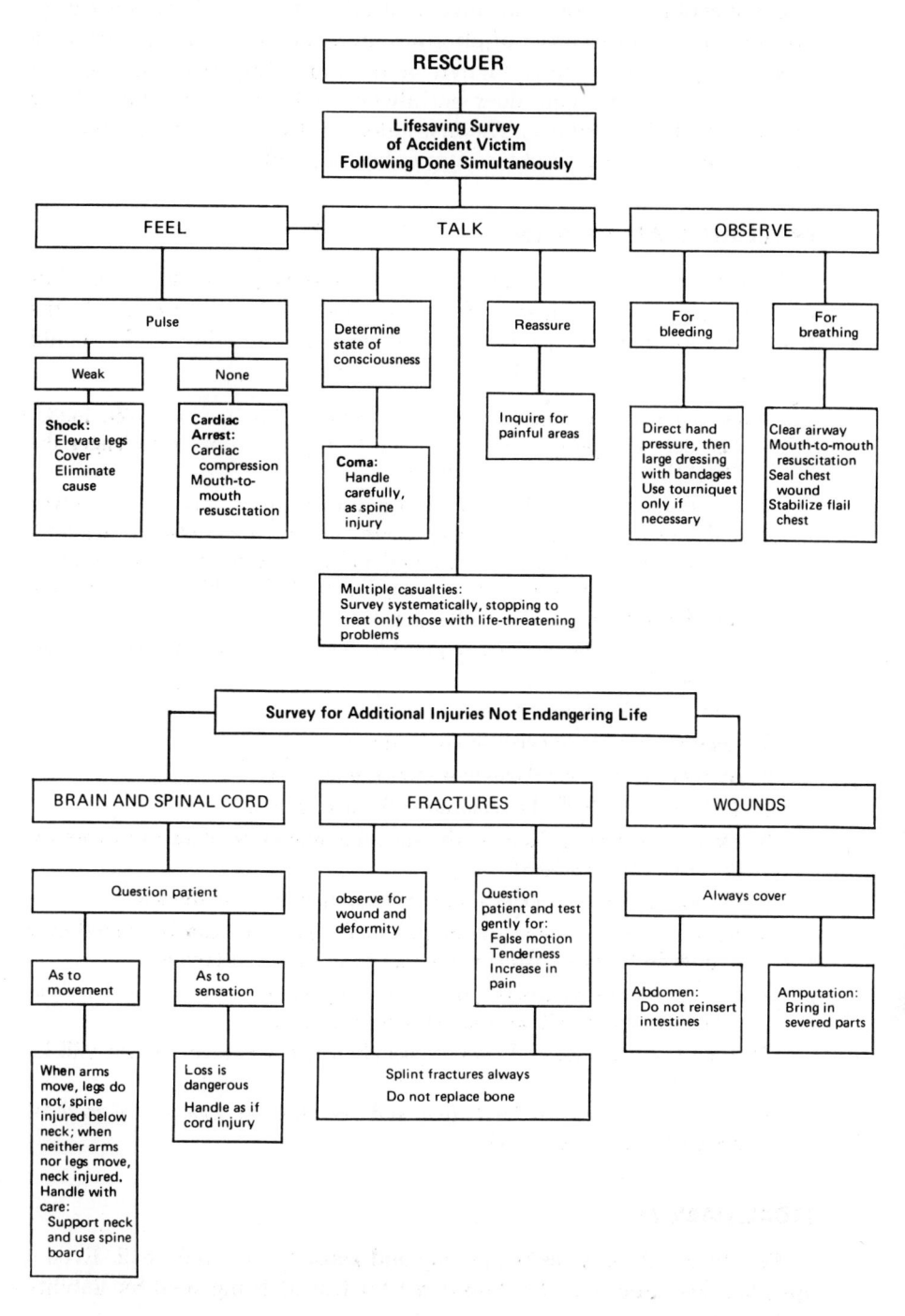

```
                              RESCUER
                                 │
                    Lifesaving Survey
                    of Accident Victim
                Following Done Simultaneously
         ┌───────────────────┼───────────────────┐
        FEEL                TALK              OBSERVE
```

FEEL
- Pulse
  - Weak → **Shock:** Elevate legs, Cover, Eliminate cause
  - None → **Cardiac Arrest:** Cardiac compression, Mouth-to-mouth resuscitation

TALK
- Determine state of consciousness
  - **Coma:** Handle carefully, as spine injury
- Reassure
  - Inquire for painful areas

OBSERVE
- For bleeding: Direct hand pressure, then large dressing with bandages. Use tourniquet only if necessary
- For breathing: Clear airway, Mouth-to-mouth resuscitation, Seal chest wound, Stabilize flail chest

Multiple casualties: Survey systematically, stopping to treat only those with life-threatening problems

Survey for Additional Injuries Not Endangering Life

BRAIN AND SPINAL CORD
- Question patient
  - As to movement: When arms move, legs do not, spine injured below neck; when neither arms nor legs move, neck injured. Handle with care: Support neck and use spine board
  - As to sensation: Loss is dangerous. Handle as if cord injury

FRACTURES
- observe for wound and deformity
- Question patient and test gently for: False motion, Tenderness, Increase in pain
- Splint fractures always. Do not replace bone

WOUNDS
- Always cover
  - Abdomen: Do not reinsert intestines
  - Amputation: Bring in severed parts

Source: American College of Surgeons. Survey developed by Sam W. Banks, M.D., F.A.C.S. and J. D. Farrington, M.D., F.A.C.S.

minor bleeding wounds, and obvious death. Of course it is not always possible to follow this order of priorities. In reality, priority depends upon locating the most seriously injured or ill, and seeing that they receive prompt, proper care. One does not always find respiratory difficulty or uncontrollable hemorrhage. The first aider must evaluate the seriousness or life-threatening aspect of the injuries he finds and act accordingly.

PROCEDURES AT THE SCENE

First aid at the scene of an injury or illness begins with action. This in itself helps both the first aider and the victim to remain calm. As the first aider proceeds to care for the most severely injured or ill, he should keep several points in mind:

1. Do not move an injured individual from the position in which found. The only exception would be where that position might endanger the life of the individual or the first aider.
2. Determine whether the individual is breathing by opening the airway and feeling for an air exchange. Also feel for the pulse at the neck (carotid) artery. If no pulse is found and there is no breathing, institute cardiopulmonary resuscitation immediately. If breathing and pulse are found, continue to maintain an open airway.
3. Protect the individual from possible harm from bystanders and surroundings.
4. Cover to help prevent shock.
5. Loosen any tight or constricting clothing.
6. Apply necessary bandages and splints, if available.
7. Talk to the individual to comfort and reassure him.
8. Do not attempt to diagnose or judge the injuries or illness; just care for the indicators exhibited.
9. Do not talk to bystanders about the condition of the individual.
10. Remain in charge until the injured or ill individual can be turned over to qualified persons, namely, police, rescue squad, or family.
11. Do not look in wallets or purses for identification. If medical identification is present it will be around the wrist or neck.
12. Keep the situation as found, especially if a police investigation will be necessary.
13. Recognize your own limitations and see that the emergency medical system has been activated.

LEGAL LIABILITY

People are often reluctant to stop and assist the injured or ill. Even a qualified first aider may hesitate to act for fear of being sued for liability

Figure 1.6 GOOD SAMARITAN STATUTES

	Date law enacted.	Covers any emergency or accident.	Covers only roadside accidents.	Covers only physicians licensed in state.	Covers out-of-state physicians.	Covers physicians and other health personnel.	Covers everyone.	Does not cover acts of gross negligence or willful misconduct.	Covers only gratuitous services.
Alabama	1966	•			•	•		•	•
Alaska	1962	•			•			•	
Arizona	1967	•				•	•	•	•
Arkansas	1963	•		•			•	•	•
Colorado	1965	•			•	•		•	
California	1959	•		•			•	•	
Connecticut	1963	•			•			•	•
Delaware	1963	•		•				•	
Florida	1965	•					•	•	•
Georgia	1962	•					•	•	•
Hawaii	1966	•					•	•	•
Idaho	1965	•				•	•	•	
Illinois	1965	•			•	•		•	
Indiana	1963	•				•		•	
Iowa	1969	•					•	•	•
Kansas	1965	•			•	•		•	•
Kentucky									
Louisiana	1964	•			•	•		•	•
Maine	1961	•				•		•	
Maryland	1963	•		•				•	•
Massachusetts	1962		•		•			•	
Michigan	1963	•			•	•		•	
Minnesota									
Mississippi	1962	•				•		•	
Missouri									
Montana	1963	•					•	•	•
Nebraska	1961	•				•		•	•
Nevada	1963	•				•		•	•
New Hampshire	1963		•		•			•	•
New Jersey	1963	•				•	•	•	
New Mexico	1963	•				•		•	•
New York	1964	•			•			•	
North Carolina	1965		•				•	•	
North Dakota	1961	•			•			•	
Ohio	1963	•					•	•	•
Oklahoma	1963	•				•	•	•	
Oregon	1967	•				•		•	•
Pennsylvania	1963	•				•	•	•	
Rhode Island	1963	•			•	•		•	
South Carolina	1964	•					•	•	•
South Dakota	1961	•			•			•	
Tennessee	1963	•					•	•	•
Texas	1961	•					•	•	•
Utah	1961	•				•		•	
Vermont									
Virginia	1962		•					•	
Virgin Islands	1964	•			•			•	•
Washington									
West Virginia	1967	•				•		•	•
Wisconsin	1963	•				•		•	
Wyoming	1961	•					•	•	•

Source: American Medical Association, AMA News Graphichart.

by the individuals he helps or by their family. This fear is generally unfounded. Court records show no case where a lay first aider, acting in good faith, assisted an ill or injured individual, and was successfully sued thereafter. Still the fear persists in the minds of many.

It may be well to remember that being a qualified first aider does not obligate you to stop and assist anyone. Only if directly responsible for the injury-causing situation are you required by law (in most states) to stop and offer assistance. Of course it is hoped that one who is trained in first aid will feel a moral obligation to help others in an emergency, without fear of legal action. Once the first aider elects to render assistance, he becomes responsible for his actions, so to minimize the possibility of suit, the first aider should:

1. Recognize and care for the life-threatening injuries or illnesses immediately.
2. Recognize his own limitations and see that the emergency medical system is activated as quickly as possible.
3. Follow recognized accepted first aid procedures when caring for an injured or ill individual.
4. Proceed to care for the individual carefully, explaining to the individual, if necessary, what is being done to assist him.

To overcome the fear of liability suits, many states have enacted Good Samaritan laws. These were designed largely to protect medical personnel (doctors, nurses, rescue squads) from suit except for gross negligence, as long as no compensation is requested. For the most part, the lay first aider is not protected by these laws (see Figure 1.6). But if he follows the points listed above and works to the best of his ability, the first aider need not be afraid of being sued. As a matter of fact, many people express their gratitude to the first aider. But the best reward is the satisfaction in having performed a helpful service and perhaps saved a life.

{ 2 }

CARDIOPULMONARY RESUSCITATION

Fatalities due to heart attack, stroke, electrocution, drowning, and head injury often do not occur as a direct result of these primary causes but as a result of *respiratory arrest*. For example, when an individual lapses into unconsciousness, his head my fall forward allowing the tongue to slide back into the throat, thereby blocking the air passage and asphyxiating him. Many lives can be saved if immediate action is taken (1) to maintain an open airway and (2) to provide artificial ventilation.

RESPIRATORY ARREST

For overcoming respiratory arrest, mouth-to-mouth resuscitation is not a new life-saving technique. A biblical reference to it appears in II Kings, where Elisha ". . . lay upon the child and put his mouth upon his mouth, his eyes upon his eyes, and his hands upon his hands, and the breath of the child waxed warm." But not until the early 1950's was this method found to be physiologically sound, and it became generally accepted as a first aid technique for laymen in 1958. Prior to the acceptance of mouth-to-mouth resuscitation, the Shaefer prone-pressure method, the Holger-Nielson back-pressure arm-lift method, and the Silvester chest-pressure arm-lift method were practiced with varying degrees of success. It has since been proven conclusively that mouth-to-mouth resuscitation is far superior to any of these former methods, and it is the choice ventilation technique.

Physiology of Respiration

Respiration is simply a gaseous exchange process. The lungs are transfer areas where oxygen is extracted from the air (normal air contains approximately 21 percent oxygen) and is absorbed directly into the blood stream. This process is known as external respiration, or *ventilation*. The blood then transports the oxygen to all tissues of the body. During this process, which is known as internal respiration, carbon dioxide is produced by the body cells as they utilize oxygen. The blood transports the carbon dioxide back to the lungs where it is then released through the exhaled air (which contains approximately 16 percent oxygen). Since oxygen cannot be stored, the average adult must breathe 12 to 20 times per minute to maintain his body demand. The respiration rate for children is slightly higher. Breathing rates are easily affected, especially by physical exertion, emotions, drugs, illness, or injury.

Thus the breathing process provides the human body with a continuous supply of oxygen. Because this continuous oxygen supply is necessary to maintain life, should it be interrupted the body will not get a fresh supply of oxygen and there will be a buildup of carbon dioxide. This resultant condition is termed *anoxia*. Within a few minutes, the vital organs (particularly the brain) may suffer permanent damage, and eventually death will occur. Figure 2.1 shows the recovery rate for resuscitation in terms of time elapsed.

Figure 2.1 RECOVERY RATES FOR RESUSCITATION

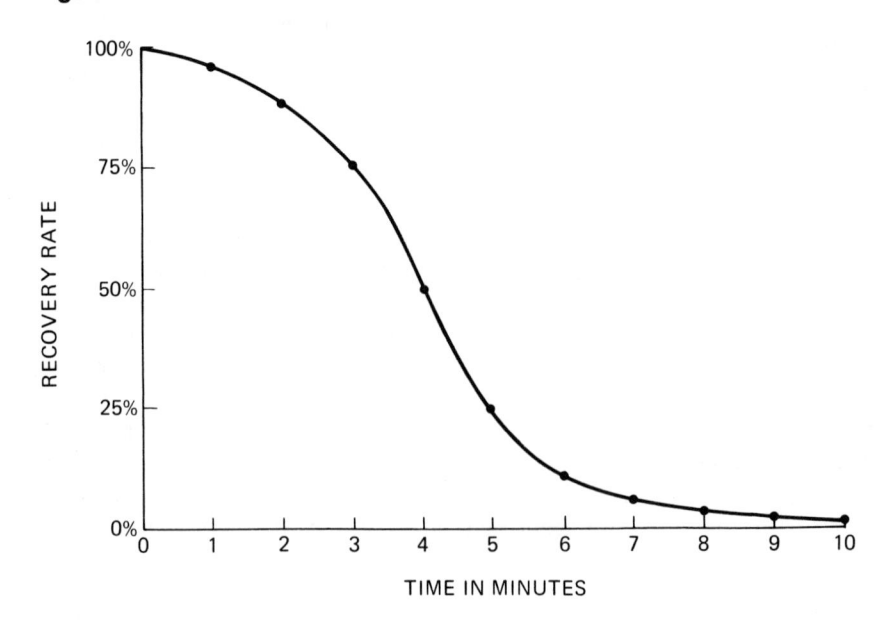

Respiratory distress may be considered in two categories: (1) airway blockage, and (2) physiological cessation of breathing.

Airway Blockage

The three principal causes of airway blockage are foreign objects, the tongue, and a form of shock called anaphylaxis.

Airway blockage occurs when foreign materials such as small toys, coins, chunks of food, mucus, vomitus, or liquids, partially or completely block the air passage. It may also occur when a person becomes unconscious, in which state his head falls forward and the muscles of the tongue and lower jaw relax, causing the jaw to sag and the base of the tongue to slide back in the throat and block the air passage. This is often erroneously referred to as "swallowing the tongue" (Figure 2.2).

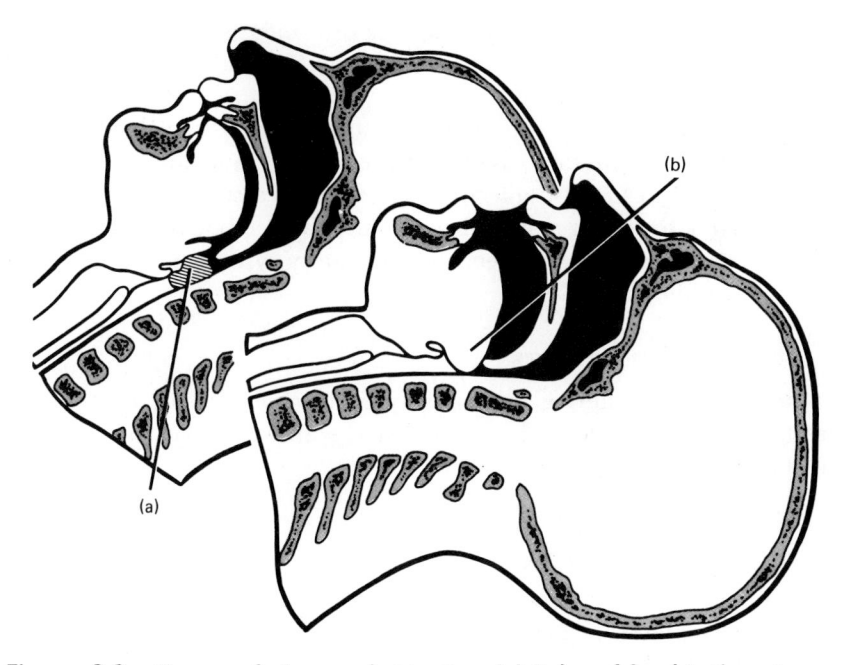

Figure 2.2 Causes of airway obstruction. (a) Bolus of food in throat. (b) Tongue in back of throat obstructing the trachea.

Anaphylaxis is a type of shock that may occur in individuals extremely sensitive to certain foods, drugs, or insect stings. The body's reaction to the allergen (sensitive agent) causes the vocal cords to swell, resulting in airway blockage. This condition is described in greater detail under Shock in Chapter 5.

Cessation of Breathing

The breathing mechanism may completely cease as a result of certain conditions affecting the nervous system, respiratory system, or circulatory system.

Injury or disease to the brain or spinal cord such as skull fractures, neck and back fractures, or brain concussions may cause an immediate cessation of the respiratory mechanism. In the same manner certain diseases which affect the brain such as meningitis, polio, or encephalitis may also cause the breathing mechanism to cease, although more slowly.

Many drugs (particularly narcotics, sleeping pills, and tranquilizers) and alcoholic beverages, especially when taken in excessive amounts or together, cause a slowing down or complete cessation of the respiratory mechanism. Likewise many toxic gases have an immediate and direct affect on the nervous system.

Direct respiratory interference such as drowning, strangulation, suffocation, smoke inhalation, choking, sucking chest wounds, broken ribs, and crushing may all cause anoxia.

A severe heart attack (cardiac arrest) affects the flow of blood to the brain, which results in the cessation of breathing. Traumatic shock, as explained in Chapter 5, also affects the circulatory system and in turn inhibits or halts breathing. Internal poisoning, carbon monoxide inhalation, and electrocution may also affect the circulatory system and cause cessation of breathing.

Indicators of Respiratory Arrest

An individual suffering from airway obstruction may or may not be breathing. This will depend on whether the airway is partially or completely obstructed.

PARTIAL AIRWAY OBSTRUCTION

1. *Gasping.* Breathing becomes a real effort.
2. *Noisy.* Snoring or garglish sound with each breath.
3. *Facial expression.* Bulging of the eyes and reddish skin color.
4. *Lightheadedness.*
5. *Dizziness.*

COMPLETE AIRWAY OBSTRUCTION

1. *Unconsciousness.* A person who has stopped breathing will be unconscious.
2. *Absence of respiratory movements.* There will be no rising and falling action of the chest. The first aider should actually *feel* for this movement, and not rely upon what he sees or thinks he sees (Figure 2.3).

Cardiopulmonary Resuscitation   [19]

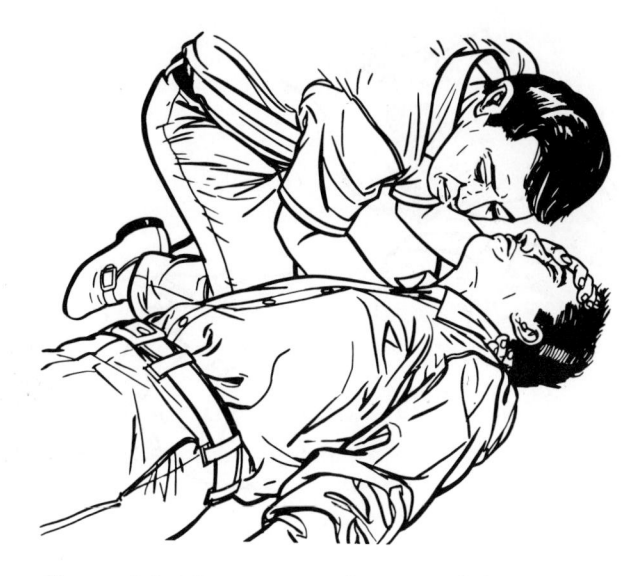

Figure 2.3 Recognition of airway obstruction.
Look, listen, and feel for air exchange.
Check for cyanosis.

3. *Lack of airflow.* Air movements into and out of the nose and mouth will have ceased—the first aider will not be able to feel or hear air movement at the nose or mouth.
4. *Cyanosis.* Facial skin will be pale or bluish, lips and fingernails also bluish in color. In dark complected individuals the first aider should check the inside of the lips, as the mucous membranes are affected rather quickly due to anoxia.
5. *Head position.* The neck may have tilted the head forward, causing the tongue to drop back and block the air passage.

ARTIFICIAL VENTILATION

There are many methods of artificial ventilation, but they all must start with the same preliminary procedure for providing an open airway so that air may get into the lungs. The procedure for clearing the airway involves two steps: positioning the victim, and positioning the victim's head.

Procedure for Opening the Airway

1. *Position the individual.*
Ideally the individual should be lying on his back, face up. In some cases, for example, in an automobile collision, the individual may have

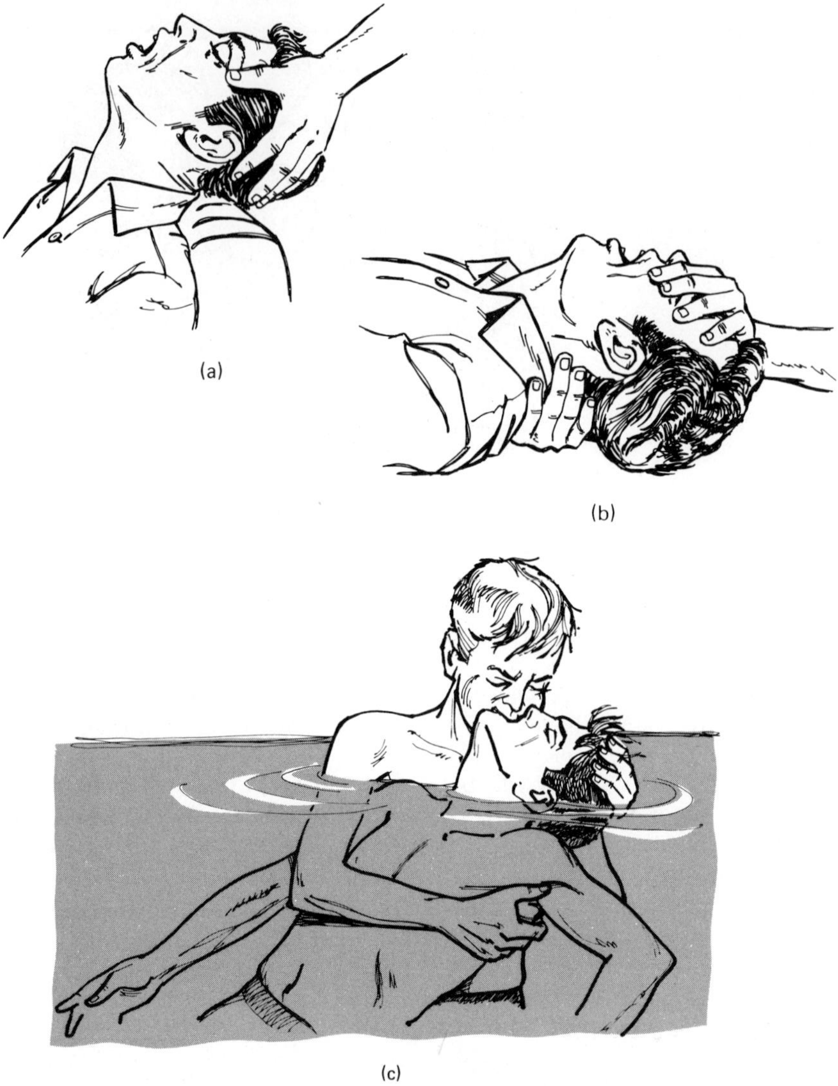

[20] Cardiopulmonary Resuscitation

Figure 2.4 Positions for open airway. An open airway may be maintained whether seated (a), lying on back (b), or in water (c).

suffered other injuries and it will not be possible to immediately place him on his back (Figure 2.4). If that is the case, leave the individual in his original position and continue with the next step.

Drowning individuals do not always have water in the lungs. Even if they do, it is impossible to remove this water so time should not be wasted in attempting to drain the lungs. Begin mouth-to-mouth resuscitation immediately. It may be possible to begin resuscitation while the victim is still in the water. When the individual has been removed from the water, check for a pulse since his heart may also have stopped. If there is no pulse present and the pupils of the eyes are dilated, begin cardiopulmonary resuscitation immediately.

2. *Position the head.*

Proper positioning of the head is the most important procedure which must be performed prior to artificial ventilation. As previously stated, an unconscious person whose head falls forward so that the chin is down may suffer anatomical blockage to the airway as a result of the tongue sliding back over the tracheal opening. This situation is easily corrected by placing the individual face up and tilting the head back (Figure 2.5a). This may be accomplished by placing one's hand under the neck, or by placing a pillow, rolled coat, or blanket under the shoulder blades (not under the head), so as to cause the head to hyperextend, that is, tilt back as far as it can. In most cases this position automatically places the tongue forward, providing an open airway. If this method fails, it may become necessary to grasp the lower jaw (Figure 2.5b) and lift the chin, tilting the head backwards. The individual is now ready to be ventilated.

There are various methods of administering artificial ventilation, and several are discussed below.

Mouth-to-Mouth

When administering mouth-to-mouth ventilation to an adult, the individual's head must be hyperextended and his mouth open. Pinching his

(a)

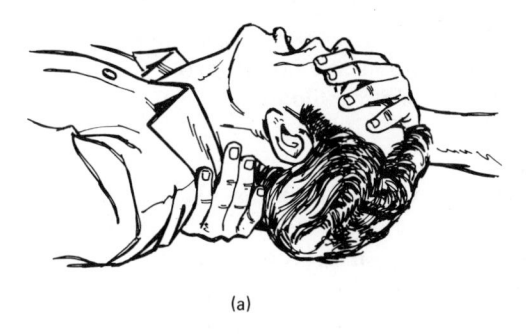

Figure 2.5 Methods of opening the airway.
(a) Tilt the head maximally backward.
(b) Lift the lower jaw upward by grasping and pulling it upward.

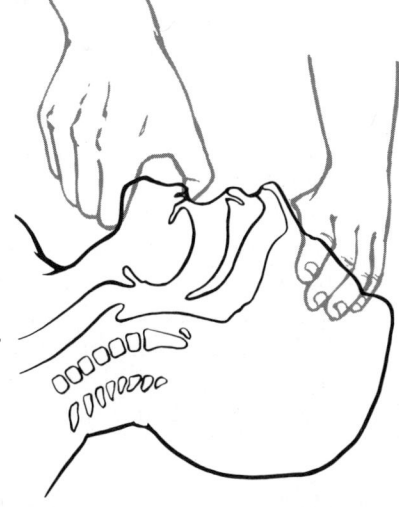

(b)

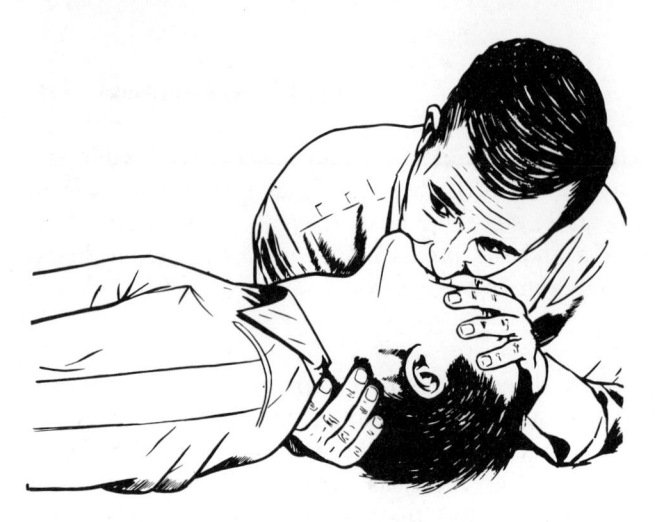

Figure 2.6 Mouth-to-mouth ventilation. Air is forced into the lungs until the chest is seen to rise.

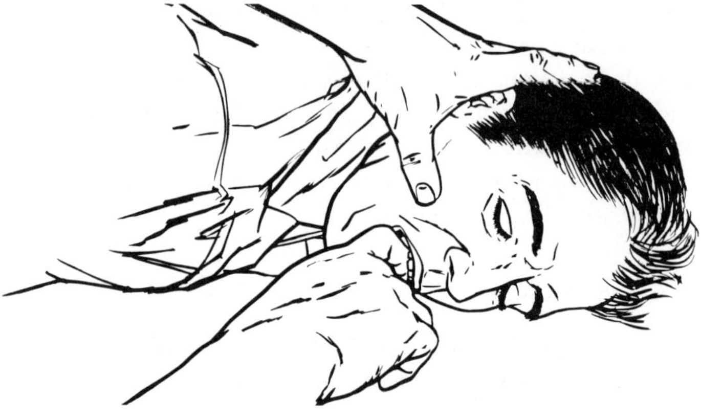

Figure 2.7 Check for airway obstruction. Clearing the airway is the first step in performing artificial ventilation.

nostrils closed, take a deep breath and completely cover his mouth with yours to create an airtight seal (Figure 2.6). Continue by exhaling into the individual's mouth until the chest inflates. Remove your mouth to allow for exhalation, at the same time turning your head to watch to see if the chest rises. If the chest rises, continue to ventilate at a rate of 12 times per minute. If it does not, air is not getting into the lungs and the first aider must check for airway obstructions.

Check to make sure that the mouth and throat are clear of foreign matter (vomitus, chewing gum, food, false teeth, etc.). Turn the individual's head to one side and with your fingers clear the mouth and throat of foreign matter (Figure 2.7). Be careful not to further block the air passage by pushing foreign matter deeper into the mouth. If foreign matter is lodged in the throat, the first aider should turn the individual on his side and administer a sharp blow to the back between the shoulder blades so as to dislodge the trapped matter (Figure 2.8a). In the case of small children, hold them securely by the feet and turn them upside down.

(a)

(b)

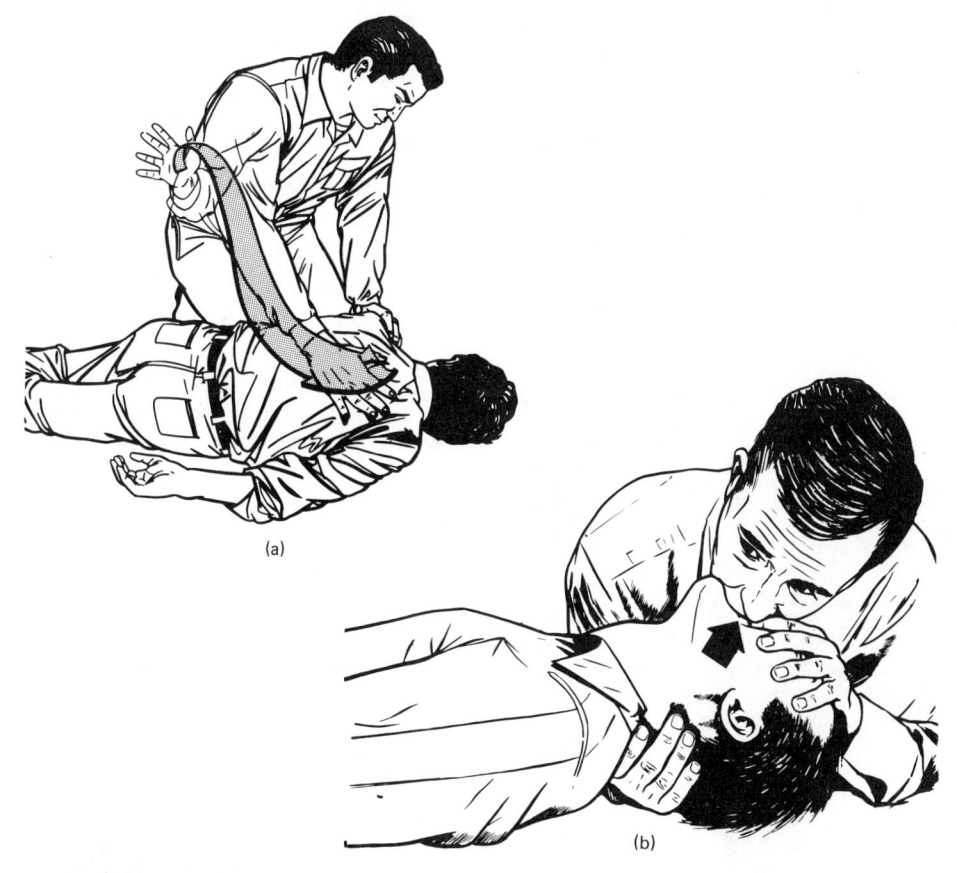

Figure 2.8 Clearing the airway. If airway is blocked, the first aider may: (a) turn the individual on his side and administer sharp slaps between the shoulder blades, or (b) perform manual suction by sucking out instead of blowing into the mouth.

Often this is sufficient to dislodge the object but if not, a sharp blow to the back may do the trick. If the object is lodged in the larynx, the previous method will not successfully dislodge it, and suction (aspiration) is required. In the absence of a mechanical aspirator, mouth-to-mouth suction

[24] Cardiopulmonary Resuscitation

should be attempted. This is accomplished by placing one's mouth over the individual's mouth and forcefully inhaling, thus producing manual suction (Figure 2.8b). For further discussion of dislodging techniques, see section on Café Coronary.

The same steps outlined for adults should be used for small children and infants, with the following exceptions: Place your mouth over the child's *mouth and nose* (Figure 2.9). Do not exhale as forcefully as with adults—just enough to cause the chest to rise. With infants, shallow puffs should be sufficient. Ventilate at the rate of 20 times per minute.

Mouth-to-Nose

Mouth-to-nose ventilation is similar to mouth-to-mouth except that the first aider exhales directly into the individual's nose instead of his mouth (Figure 2.10). This method is used when injuries or immovable obstructions are present in the mouth or when clenched jaws prevent using the mouth as an airway. When administering mouth-to-nose ventilation it is

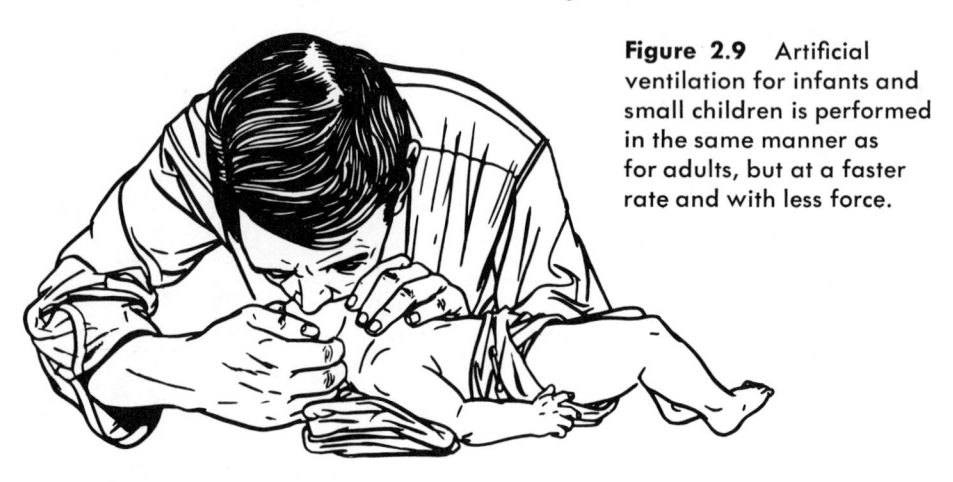

Figure 2.9 Artificial ventilation for infants and small children is performed in the same manner as for adults, but at a faster rate and with less force.

Figure 2.10 Mouth-to-nose ventilation.

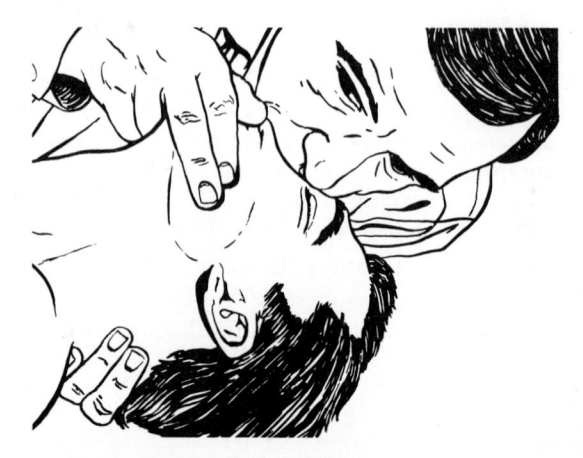

AIRWAY   S-TUBE

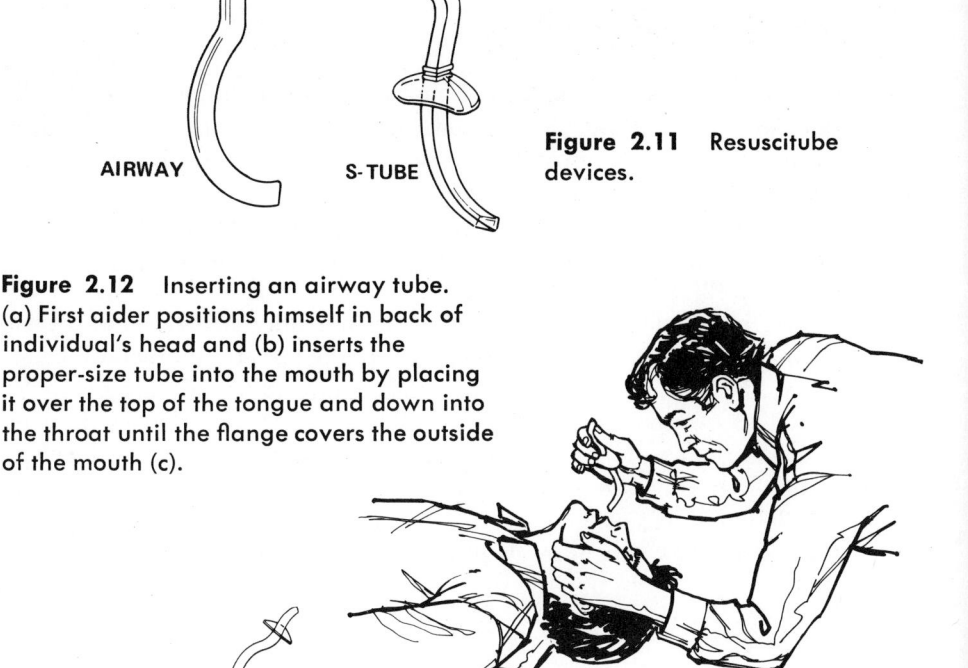

Figure 2.11 Resuscitube devices.

Figure 2.12 Inserting an airway tube. (a) First aider positions himself in back of individual's head and (b) inserts the proper-size tube into the mouth by placing it over the top of the tongue and down into the throat until the flange covers the outside of the mouth (c).

important to hold the individual's mouth tightly closed with one hand to prevent air leakage. After exhaling into the nose, allow the individual's mouth to open for exhalation. Special attention must be paid to see that the jaw is maximally extended upward.

Mouth-to-Airway (Resuscitube)

The unique feature of resuscitube devices (see Figure 2.11) is that a tube is inserted into the individual's throat and the first aider breaths into the tube to aid in the maintenance of an open airway. The devices come in adult, child, and infant sizes. But no airway tubes of any kind should ever be used unless the first aider has been properly trained and is totally familiar with their use. Furthermore, airway tubes should be used only if the individual is *un*conscious, because in a conscious person the gag reflex interferes with inserting the tube.

As with all mouth-to-mouth techniques, the individual should be on his back with his head hyperextended. To insert an airway properly (Figure 2.12), the first aider positions himself in back of the individual's head. He inserts the proper-size tube into the individual's mouth, placing it over the top of the tongue and down into the throat until the oval flange covers the outside of the mouth. Using his index fingers, the first aider firmly presses the flange down against the mouth and pinches the nose with his thumbs to prevent air from escaping. Care must be taken to maintain the hyperextended position of the head. As mouth-to-airway ventilation is administered, watch for chest movements. Continue ventilations at the same rate as for mouth-to-mouth, described above.

Bag-Mask Resuscitation

The bag-mask device is often carried by ambulance and rescue squad crews and is relatively simple to use. The unit consists of a plastic or rubberized balloon with a face mask attached to one end. The first aider uses one hand to hold the mask down firmly over the individual's mouth and nose (Figure 2.13), and with the other hand squeezes the oval-shaped bag to force air into the individual's lungs. As always, it is important to keep the head hyperextended in order to maintain an open airway. If available, an airway tube should be inserted into the individual's throat in the same manner as a resuscitube. Bag-mask resuscitators come with detachable masks, usually two sizes, adult and child. They are equipped with a valve which prevents the individual from exhaling into the bag. Most units are designed so that oxygen can also be piped into the bag.

Figure 2.13 Bag-mask ventilation.

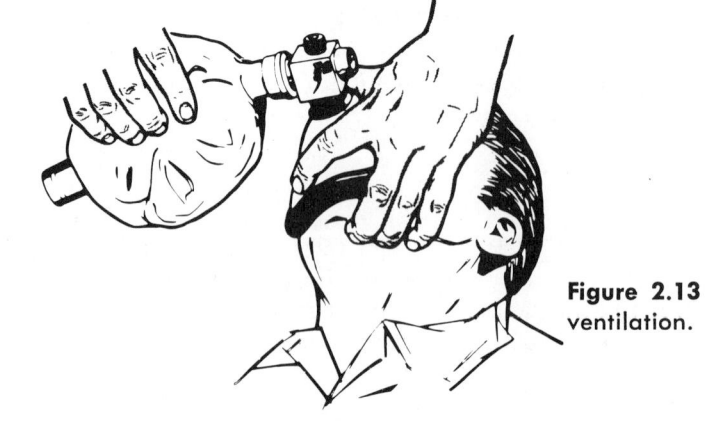

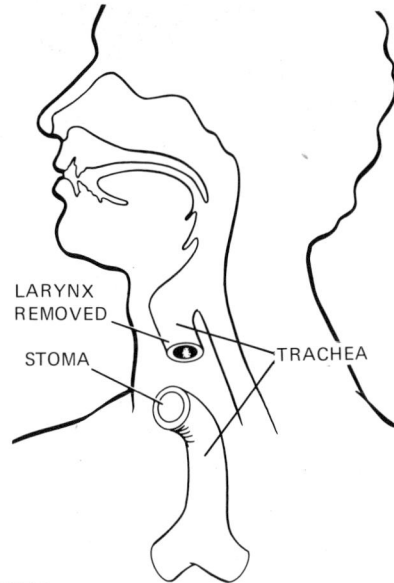

Figure 2.14 Anatomy of a laryngectomee.

Mouth-to-Stoma

A laryngectomee is a person who has had his vocal chords and outer portion of the larynx removed. In this case the trachea is brought through an opening in the front of the neck. This opening is called a stoma and its purpose is to provide a new airway into the lungs (Figure 2.14). Laryngectomees do not breathe through the mouth and nose but through the stoma. At times it is difficult to recognize a laryngectomee immediately as the stoma may be covered by clothing, jewelry, or a piece of gauze which acts as a dust filter.

Not all laryngectomees have achieved speech and those that have find it hard to speak after eating or while lying down. Also, some laryngectomees wear a tracheotomy tube, which is usually held in place with a chain or a band around the neck. This tube must be cleaned before mouth-to-stoma ventilation can be started. Carefully remove the tube and clean it. Be certain that the stoma is also clear, then gently reinsert the tube. Mouth-to-stoma resuscitation can now be started. This form of resuscitation is similar to mouth-to-mouth except that the first aider breathes directly into the stoma. To provide greater accessibility to the stoma, it is advisable to place the individual on his back with a pillow or similar object under his shoulders. The first aider then places his mouth firmly over the stoma and proceeds as with mouth-to-mouth resuscitation (Figure 2.15).

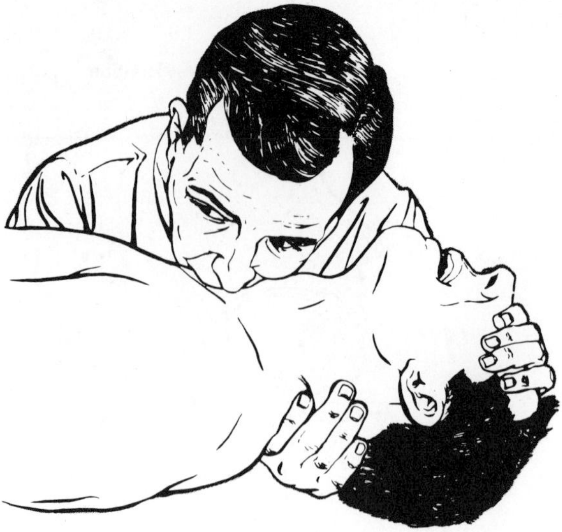

Figure 2.15 Mouth-to-stoma ventilation.

Indicators of Effective Ventilation

If air is entering the body effectively, the first aider will see the chest rise. In addition, skin color begins to return to normal and spontaneous breathing may occur. However, even if the individual does begin to breathe, he must be observed carefully, because arrest may reoccur. If the chest does not rise upon blowing into the mouth, there may be a foreign-body obstruction, improper head position, or laryngectomee situation.

CAFÉ CORONARY

A special type of respiratory obstruction known as the *café coronary*, has received a good deal of attention recently. It has been found that many deaths from apparent heart attack are actually caused by airway obstruction from food stuck in the trachea. The typical situation involves an individual, usually wearing dentures and having had a few cocktails, who attempts to swallow solid food. The individual is suddenly unable to talk, groan, cough, or breathe. He collapses and within minutes dies from an apparent heart attack. Autopsies performed on this type of sudden death often find large pieces of food lodged in the trachea. Apparently these individuals, because of ill-fitting or absent dentures, have fallen into the habit of swallowing large pieces of food, and under the influence of alcohol, attempt to swallow a big chunk which won't go down and blocks the airway.

Care for the Café Coronary

There are three methods of assisting an individual with food obstructing the airway: (1) pull the food out of the throat with one's fingers, (2) use a device known as a Choke-Saver,* and (3) pop the food out by the "Heimlich maneuver."†

Initially the first aider should open the victim's mouth and if he can see the obstructing piece of food, reach into the mouth with his middle and index fingers and pull the food out. Care must be taken not to push the food deeper into the throat.

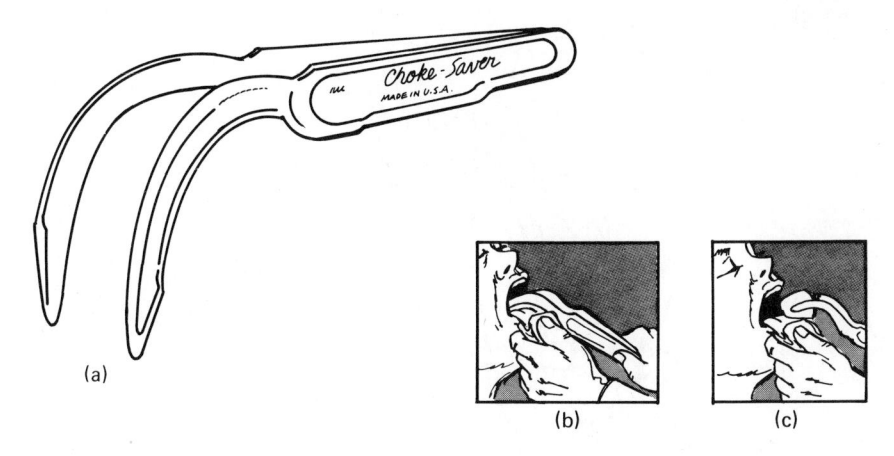

Figure 2.16 The Choke-Saver device is used to remove food obstructions from the throat.

If this procedure is unsuccessful, the Choke-Saver may be used if available. This device is being placed in restaurants and other public places where food is consumed. Designed for use by the layman, the device is a tweezer-like tongs made of plastic (Figure 2.16a). The first aider begins by tilting back the head of the victim and pulling the tongue forward. He can then easily insert the device by sliding it, in open position, along the curve of the tongue into the back of the victim's throat (Figure 2.16b). When completely inserted with the tips straddling the obstructing food, the handles are squeezed together tightly, gripping the food with the tips of the device. Maintaining this grip, the first aider then slides the Choke-Saver back over the tongue and removes it with the obstruction (Figure 2.16c). If the victim does not resume breathing spontaneously, mouth-to-mouth ventilations may be necessary and the individual should be transported to a medical facility as quickly as possible.

Some physicians have expressed concern about the use of the Choke-Saver by untrained persons. If improperly inserted the device can indeed

*Registered trademark, Dyna-Med, Inc., Leucadia, California.
†Developed by Dr. Henry J. Heimlich, Jewish Hospital, Cincinnati, Ohio.

(a)

(b)

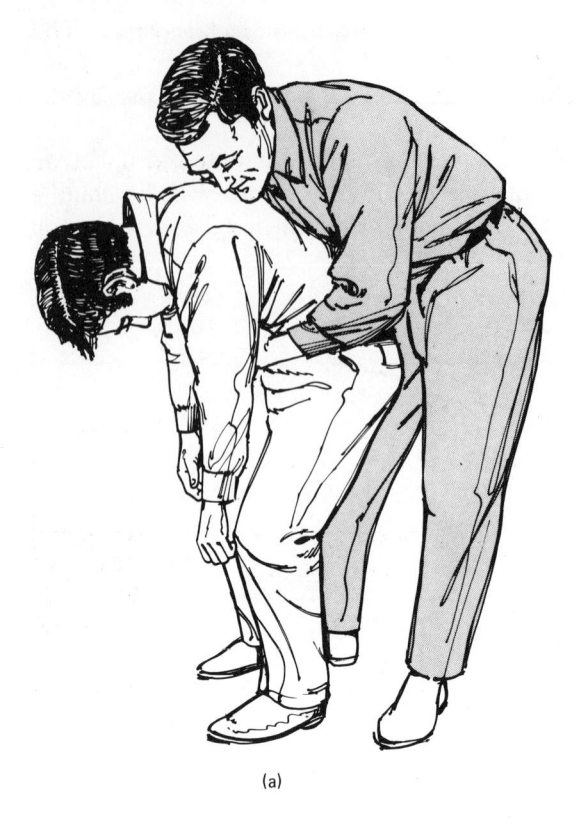

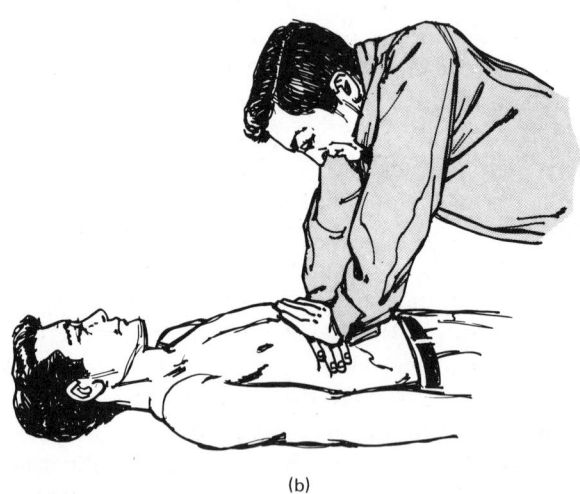

Figure 2.17 In the Heimlich maneuver, air within the victim's lungs is used to help pop the obstruction loose by pressing on the abdomen. (a) in standing position, from behind; (b) if victim is found lying face up.

bruise the throat, but the device has been designed so as to prevent or minimize serious injury to the throat tissue.

If a Choke-Saver is not available, another removal method recently developed by Dr. Henry J. Heimlich may be attempted. The Heimlich maneuver uses the remaining air within the victim's lungs to pop out the obstructing food. Standing behind the victim, the first aider places both of his arms around the victim just below the ribs, allowing the victim's head and upper body to slump forward (Figure 2.17a). He then presses rapidly and strongly into the victim's abdominal cavity forcing the diaphragm upward, causing the lungs to compress and forcefully expell the obstructing object. If the victim is found lying face up, the first aider may use both of his hands (one on top of the other) to forcefully press the abdominal cavity (just below the ribs) to obtain the same effect (Figure 2.17b). A second first aider should be ready to retrieve the ejected piece of food from the mouth of the victim. If the victim does not begin to breathe spontaneously, mouth-to-mouth ventilations may be necessary and the individual should be transported to a medical facility as quickly as possible.

If none of the three methods described succeeds in freeing the obstructed airway, the individual should be rushed by ambulance to a hospital, where an emergency tracheotomy may have to be performed in order to save his life.

HYPERVENTILATION

Hyperventilation, a fairly common reaction, is often confused by the first aider with respiratory obstruction or heart attack. The hyperventilating individual appears to have difficulty getting his breath. Although he is gasping for air, physiologically his respiratory system is suffering from too much rather than not enough oxygen. Although the body demands oxygen to survive, a certain level of carbon dioxide must be maintained in the brain in order to stimulate respiration. In hyperventilation, the carbon dioxide level in the brain is too low, so the individual needs carbon dioxide, not oxygen, as he would for respiratory failure or heart attack.

Indicators of Hyperventilation

Individuals who are prone to nervousness, anxiety, or emotional excitement are susceptible to hyperventilation when placed in a stressful situation. This condition is often seen in inexperienced athletes. The individual appears to be nervous, anxious, excited, has undergone a period of shallow

[32] Cardiopulmonary Resuscitation

rapid breathing, often undetected, exhibits difficulty breathing, and may complain of tingling or numbness in his fingers and toes. Also characteristic of hyperventilation is an ulnar deviation (wrist turned outward), with the fingers hyperextended or in a state of uncontrollable flexing. As the condition progresses, the individual may lose consciousness.

First Aid Procedures for Hyperventilation

The first aid consists of calming the individual and providing carbon dioxide to the body. This may be achieved by various methods:

1. Instruct the individual to hold his breath.
2. Instruct the individual to breathe slowly, pausing between breaths.
3. Place the individual's hands, tent fashion, over his mouth and nose and instruct him to breathe slowly into his hands. He is now re-breathing his own expired air containing the needed carbon dioxide.
4. Place a paper bag, football helmet, bowl, or similar object over the individual's mouth and nose and instruct him to breathe slowly into it. This accomplishes re-breathing to obtain the necessary carbon dioxide.
5. If the individual loses consciousness, this will in effect help to slow breathing and return the body to a more normal oxygen–carbon dioxide relationship.
6. Seek medical attention if condition persists for any length of time. It is possible that an organic or emotional problem is present which must be diagnosed and treated by a physician.

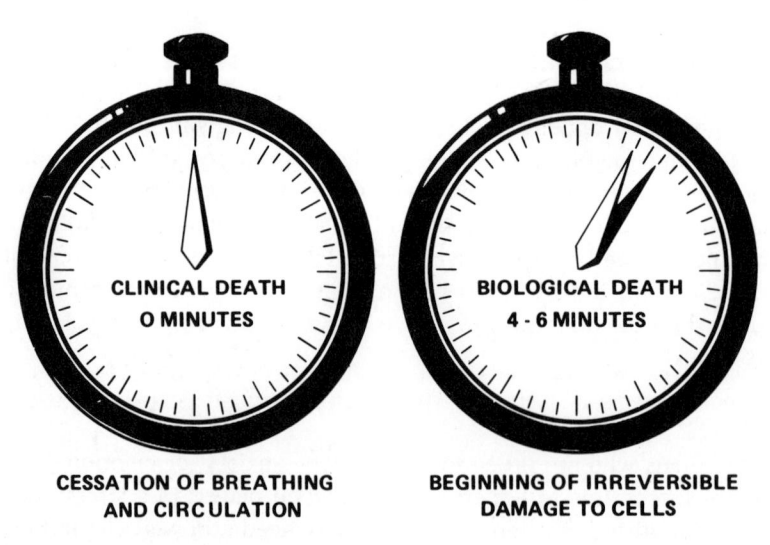

Figure 2.18 Clinical and biological death.

CARDIAC ARREST

Annually 700,000 Americans die of heart attacks. Of this number, approximately 7,500 to 9,000 die of cardiac arrest (standstill of the heart), which might have been a temporary reversible condition had the proper resuscitative techniques been applied quickly enough. Just as it is possible to revive a drowned person with mouth-to-mouth resuscitation, it is also possible to give the heart a second chance by means of cardiac massage—a method of external heart compression. Cardiac arrest may occur as a result of a heart attack, drowning, electrical shock, strangulation, suffocation, or a drug reaction. The first aider most often does not know the true condition of the heart, which can only be determined by an electrocardiogram (EKG). However, certain external indicators will be present which will indicate that cardiopulmonary resuscitation (CPR) is necessary if the individual is to live.

Physiology of Circulation

When an individual stops breathing, the heart may continue circulating blood for up to 4 to 6 minutes, depending upon the individual and the condition of his body. However, when the heart stops, breathing ceases immediately or within 30 seconds. The body remains biologically alive for about 4 to 6 minutes following cardiac arrest. The vital centers of the brain are irreversibly affected in about 4 minutes due to a lack of oxygen (Figure 2.18). In order to revive an individual, cardiopulmonary resuscitation techniques must be initiated within this 4-minute grace period, otherwise severe brain damage will occur and the individual may not function normally even though revived. If the first aider is in doubt as to how long the individual has been without oxygen, he should immediately begin CPR, transport to a hospital, and let a physician determine whether cardiopulmonary resuscitation should be continued or stopped.

Indicators of Cardiac Arrest

Cardiac massage needs to be given much less frequently than mouth-to-mouth resuscitation. The victim of cardiac arrest will exhibit those indicators of respiratory arrest which have been previously described. In addition, no pulse will be felt at the carotid (neck) artery (Figure 2.19). Within 45 seconds to one minute after circulation ceases the pupils of the eye begin to dilate, and within two minutes the eyes are completely dilated and fixed (Figure 2.20). This means that when light is shined into the eye the pupil will not constrict. The first aider should be sure to check both eyes, as the individual may have suffered a stroke or concus-

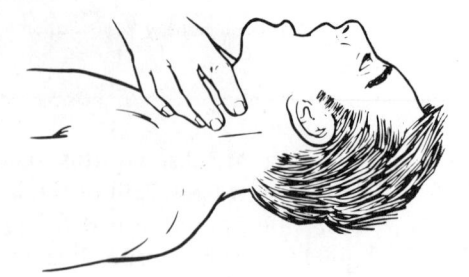

Figure 2.19 Checking for carotid pulse. In cardiac arrest no pulse will be felt.

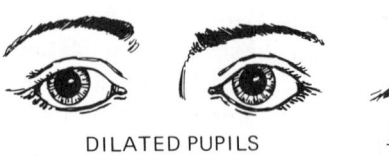

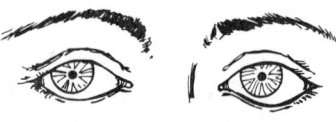

DILATED PUPILS

CONSTRICTED PUPILS

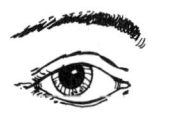

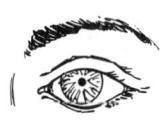

UNEQUAL PUPILS

Figure 2.20 Dilated/Constricted pupils. In cardiac arrest the eyes will be dilated as opposed to constricted or unequal.

sion, or may have an artificial eye. Fixed and dilated eyes are an indicator of cardiac arrest, along with the absence of a carotid pulse, but should not to be used as a sole indicator.

CARDIAC MASSAGE (External Heart Compression)

Cardiac massage is a method of resuscitation performed by external, manual compression of the heart, whereby the heart is rhythmically squeezed between the sternum and vertebrae until its action is restored. The technique requires knowing where to place the hands, how to exert the right pressure, and what rhythm to maintain. The technique works by compression and relaxation. Externally applied pressure forces blood out of the heart; when the pressure is released, the heart refills with blood passively (Figure 2.21). The procedure is as follows:

1. Place the individual face up on a hard surface such as the floor (cardiac massage is ineffective on a soft surface), or put a board or other hard object under the entire back.
2. Kneel at right angles to the individual's sternum (longitudinal breastbone).
3. Extend the neck to open the airway and ventilate the individual. This

Cardiopulmonary Resuscitation   [35]

step must be performed simultaneously—preferably by an additional first aider—throughout the massage.

4. Locate the pressure point—the exact point on the sternum where pressure must be applied to be effective. To find it, locate the xiphoid process at the lower end of the sternum where the sternum meets the abdominal cavity. Come up about 1 to 1½ inches from the end of the xiphoid process (toward the victim's head) and place the heel of one hand. This is the precise point for applying pressure (Figure 2.22).

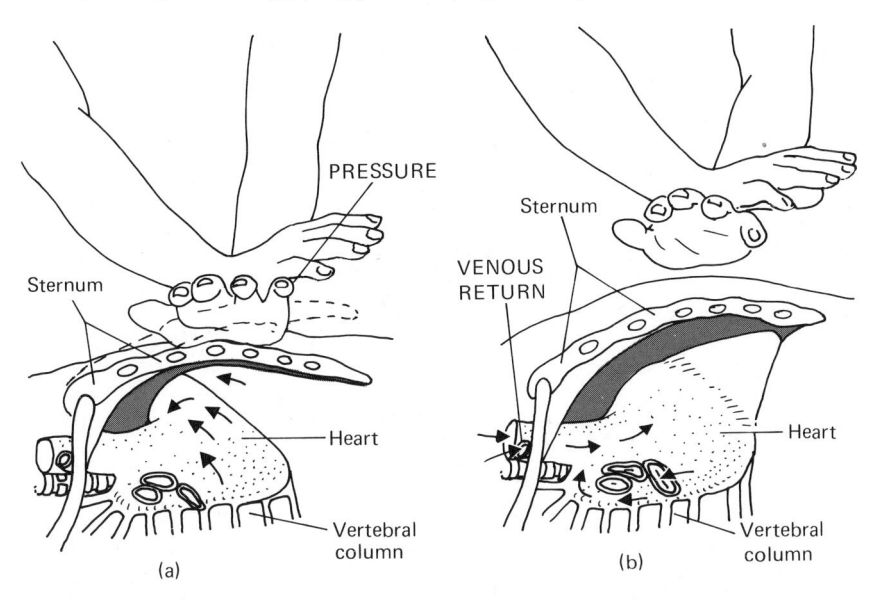

Figure 2.21 Closed heart massage consists of two phases: (a) compression, which forces the blood out of the heart, and (b) relaxation, which allows the heart to fill passively.

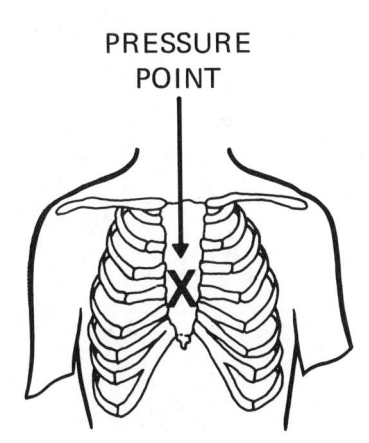

Figure 2.22 The pressure point for closed chest heart massage is located one inch above the xiphoid process on the sternum.

[36] Cardiopulmonary Resuscitation

5. Keeping the heel of one hand on the pressure point, place the other hand on top of the first. The fingers may be interlocked. Now bring your shoulders directly over the victim's sternum, keeping your arms straight, and begin to exert pressure (Figure 2.23). Pressure should be applied in a firm, smooth manner so that the sternum moves about 1½ to 2 inches downward toward the vertebrae with each thrust.
6. Release the pressure of the hands completely. This will allow the chest to expand and the heart to fill with oxygenated blood. Do not lose contact with the sternum—just relax the pressure which has been exerted.
7. Continue cardiac massage at a rate of one compression per second or 60 per minute. A rhythm of less than 60 per minute is ineffective; from 60 to about 80 is more beneficial, but if compressions are repeated too

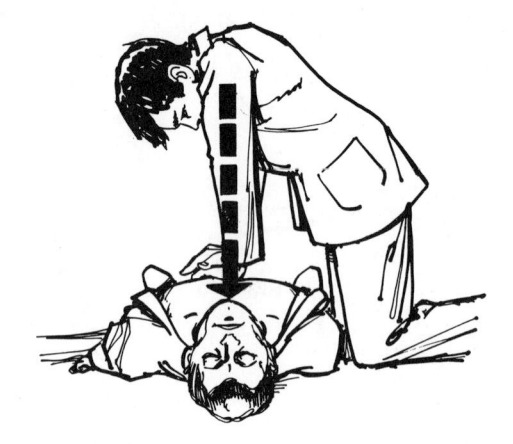

Figure 2.23 Proper positioning for performing cardiac massage on an adult.

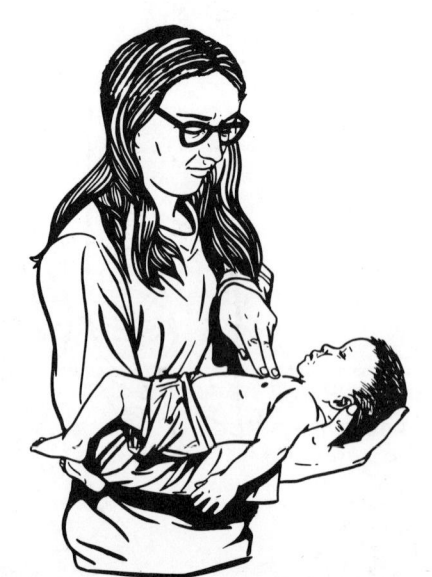

Figure 2.24 Cardiac massage for an infant.

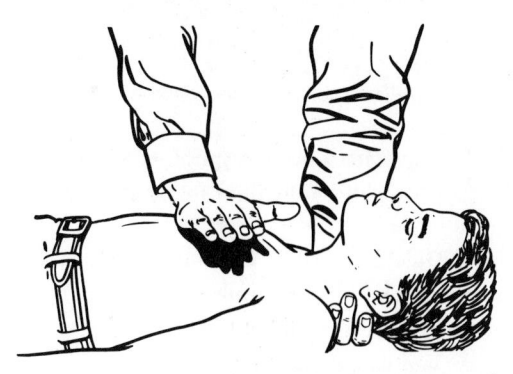

Figure 2.25 Cardiac massage for a small child.

quickly the heart will not have time to relax and fill with the oxygenated blood needed for circulation and maintenance of cell tissues. Once the rhythm is started it should not be interrupted for more than five seconds; even this slight pause may greatly reduce the individual's oxygen supply.

8. When performing external heart compression on children, the rate and pressure exerted must be modified. Children should be resuscitated at between 80 to 100 compressions per minute. Modification of pressure is even more important. If too much pressure is exerted, serious complications could result. For infants and small children, use only the tips of the fingers of one hand to the center of the sternum (Figure 2.24). For older children, up to age 9 or 10, use only the heel of one hand (Figure 2.25). The other hand can be used to provide firm pressure under the child's back.

CPR with One First Aider

If the first aider is alone and must perform both mouth-to-mouth resuscitation and external heart compression, he proceeds as follows (Figure 2.26):

Figure 2.26 Cardiopulmonary resuscitation is performed by one first aider at a ratio of 15 compressions to 2 ventilations, with a total of 80 compressions per minute.

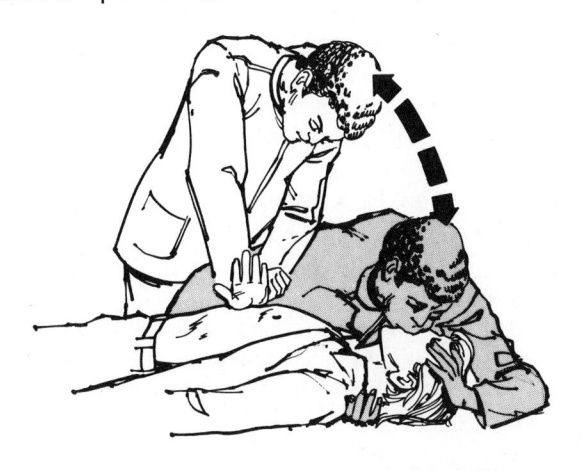

[38] Cardiopulmonary Resuscitation

1. Check for signs of respiratory movement.
2. Ready the individual for ventilation and compression as previously discussed.
3. Quickly ventilate the individual four times.
4. Check for carotid pulse and dilated pupils.
5. Compress the heart fifteen times.
6. Ventilate the individual twice.
7. Continue alternating ventilations and compressions at a ratio of 2 ventilations to 15 compressions, completing 80 compressions within one minute.
8. Seek medical attention as rapidly as possible.

CPR with Two First Aiders

If two first aiders are present, proceed as follows (Figure 2.27):

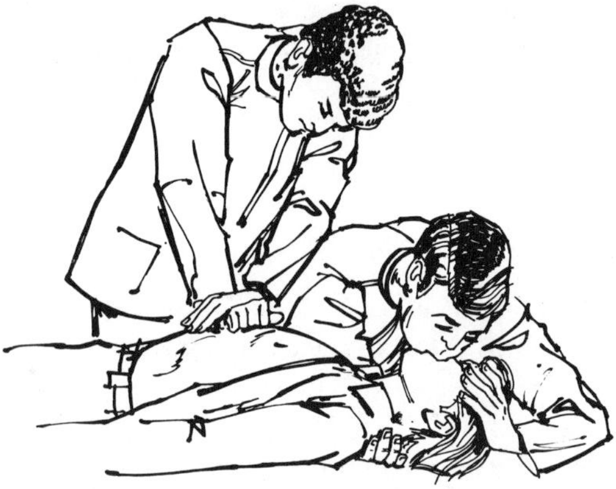

Figure 2.27 Cardiopulmonary resuscitation is performed by two first aiders at a ratio of 5 compressions to 1 ventilation, with 60 compressions completed per minute.

1. Check for signs of respiratory movements.
2. Ready the individual for ventilation and compression as previously discussed.
3. One first aider ventilates the individual four times.
4. Check for carotid pulse and dilated pupils.
5. The second first aider begins compressions at a normal rate of one per second. (In order to be coordinated with the ventilations, it helps if the first aider giving the compressions counts aloud.) After the fifth compression, one ventilation is given. This takes a bit of coordination, as the breath must be forced in between compressions to be effective.

6. Continue alternating ventilations and compressions at a ratio of 1 ventilation to 5 compressions, completing 60 compressions per minute.
7. Seek medical attention as rapidly as possible.

Summary of Cardiopulmonary Resuscitation

To help the first aider understand the sequence of procedures for performing cardiopulmonary resuscitation correctly, a decision chart has been developed. Figure 2.28 illustrates in a step-by-step manner the procedures to be followed by a first aider when he encounters an unconscious individual. First, he must check for indications of breathing. If the victim is breathing he can then check further for a pulse. If both breathing and circulation are present, the first aider continues to examine the individual for signs of injuries or illness and gives the indicated care. If there is no breathing, the first aider must first open the airway. This in itself may be sufficient to restore normal breathing. If, however, spontaneous breathing does not occur, he must begin ventilating for the victim with four full breaths. He then checks for a pulse and if none is found, continues with the standard procedures for cardiopulmonary resuscitation.

Indicators of Effective Resuscitation

Resuscitation techniques should be continued until the individual shows signs of revival or is pronounced dead by a physician. If the resuscitation techniques are successful the dilated pupils of the eyes will begin to constrict and a carotid pulse can be felt with each compression. In addition, normal skin color will begin to return. Although spontaneous breathing may occur, this is not likely. The individual will need supportive medical treatment before breathing and circulation return to normal.

Dangers of Improper Cardiac Massage

Until recently, cardiac massage was considered a medical procedure, in view of the possible complications when it is performed incorrectly. Repeated practice has shown, however, that if the techniques are taught and performed properly, external heart compression need not be hazardous. Conversely, of course, if performed improperly, damage may result (Figure 2.29).

Rib fractures of costal-cartilage separations are injuries that sometimes cannot be avoided when performing CPR effectively. This type of injury will heal easily, and is a small price to pay in saving a person's life. To

Figure 2.28 SEQUENCE OF PROCEDURES IN PERFORMING CARDIOPULMONARY RESUSCITATION

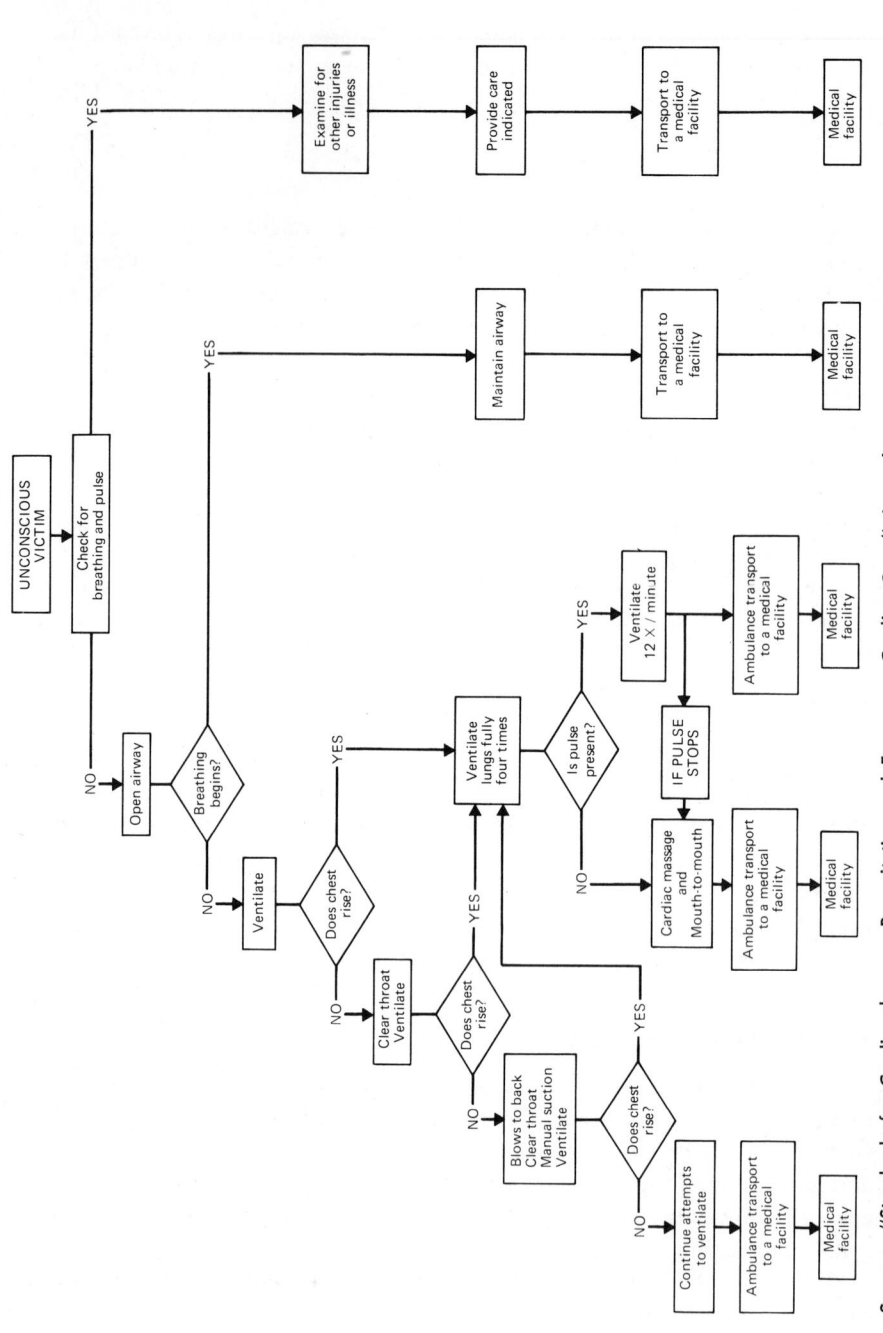

Source: "Standards for Cardiopulmonary Resuscitation and Emergency Cardiac Care," *Journal of the American Medical Association*, February 18, 1974.

Cardiopulmonary Resuscitation [41]

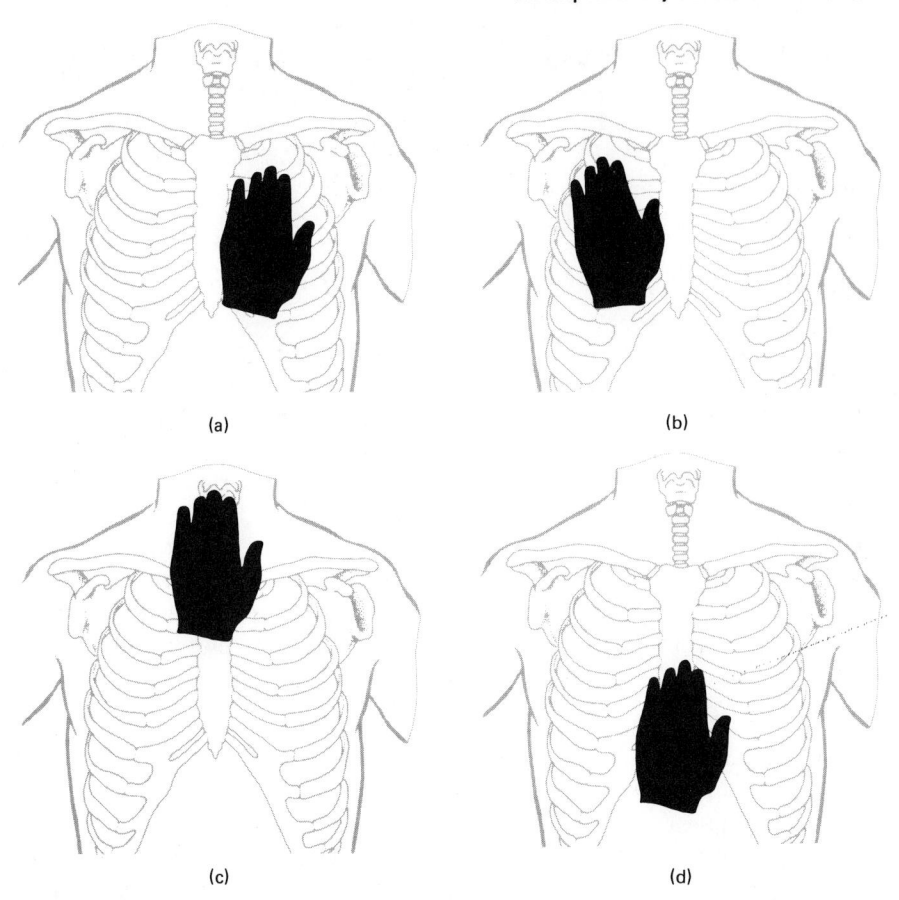

Figure 2.29 Improper cardiac massage. If the hands are too far to the left of the sternum (a) or too far to the right (b) ribs may fracture or separate from the sternum and cause lacerations to the lungs. If the hands are too high (c) there is no effective action on the heart; if too low (d) the xiphoid may break off and lacerate the liver.

lessen the possibility of fracturing the rib cage, the first aider should be careful to keep only the heel of one hand on the lower third of the sternum and keep all fingers off the ribs. The most serious complication of external heart compression is lacerations to the liver, which may come about as a result of the hands being placed too low over the xiphoid process, an area that is vulnerable to breakage or separation. It is imperative that the first aider keep his hands in the proper position on the sternum.

When properly performed, external heart compression has proven its effectiveness in cases of cardiac arrest. It provides sufficient circulation

[42] Cardiopulmonary Resuscitation

to supply body tissue with oxygen and maintain the heart and brain until the heart can resume beating on its own. It must be remembered, however, that external heart compression is ineffective unless mouth-to-mouth ventilation is performed simultaneously, and CPR is most effective when performed by two first aiders in tandem.

WITNESSED CARDIAC ARREST

There are times when a first aider will be with an individual who suddenly collapses from a cardiac arrest. In this situation if the first aider acts quickly, he may reverse the heart's nonpumping condition (ventricular fibrillation) and restore normal circulation and breathing. This is accomplished by administering a precordial thump. A precordial thump is a sharp blow to the mid-portion of the sternum to stimulate a potentially reactive heart. To be effective, however, this technique must be performed within the first minute of arrest. After that time the heart suffers from anoxia and is unable to react to this procedure. At present the precordial thump may not be used by first aiders on children.

When a first aider witnesses a cardiac arrest, the following procedures should be followed:

1. Maximally extend the head to open the airway, and simultaneously feel for a carotid pulse.
2. If no pulse is found, perform the precordial thump by giving a sharp, quick, single blow to the mid-portion of the sternum. The sternum is

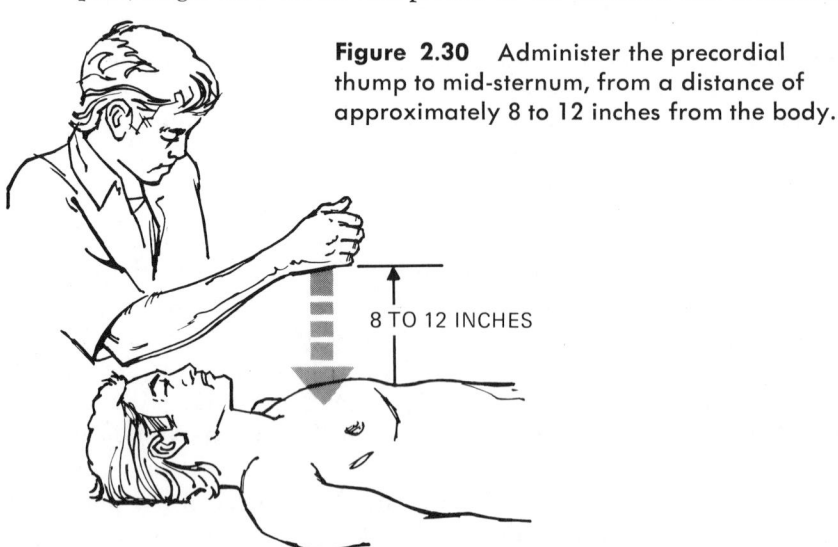

Figure 2.30 Administer the precordial thump to mid-sternum, from a distance of approximately 8 to 12 inches from the body.

8 TO 12 INCHES

hit with the bottom fleshy part of the closed fist from a distance of 8 to 12 inches (Figure 2.30).
3. If no pulse is found following the precordial thump (the precordial thump is only attempted once), continue by giving four quick full breaths, and massage the heart following the standard procedures for performing cardiopulmonary resuscitation with one or two first aiders.

INITIATING AND TERMINATING CARDIOPULMONARY RESUSCITATION

First aiders are often concerned about when to start and at what point to stop applying the life-saving skills of cardiopulmonary resuscitation. Whenever a first aider encounters an individual who has neither pulse nor breathing, the first aider should initiate cardiopulmonary resuscitation immediately. If the victim has been without oxygen for more than ten minutes or has suffered severe damage to brain or heart, resuscitative efforts are usually not effective. But since the first aider has no way of determining how long the victim has been without oxygen, he should initiate cardiopulmonary resuscitation in any case.

Cardiopulmonary resuscitation may be terminated by the first aider under any of the following circumstances:

1. The victim begins effective spontaneous circulation and ventilation—breathing and pulse return.
2. An ambulance or mobile coronary unit arrives to take over from the first aider. These units will continue resuscitative efforts until the individual reaches a medical facility. The physician at the medical facility will determine whether the resuscitative efforts are to be continued further.
3. The first aider is totally exhausted and unable to continue performing cardiopulmonary resuscitation.

{ 3 }

HEMORRHAGE CONTROL

Minor lacerations and the hemorrhage which results are among the principal types of injuries that individuals suffer and that first aiders are asked to handle. In most instances these injuries are not serious, and simple bandaging controls the bleeding. However, massive hemorrhage can occur as a result of serious injury or illness, and the first aider may encounter a life-threatening situation.

Often a hemorrhage appears far more serious than it really is, especially to first aiders who have not handled many open wounds. Not until the wound is thoroughly examined can the seriousness of the hemorrhage be determined. The extent of hemorrhage depends upon the type of injury sustained—whether a knife or gunshot wound or blunt object injury—and the part of the body and blood vessels that have been injured. For example, a knife wound in the trunk of the body that has severed arteries and lacerated vital organs is going to present a more serious hemorrhage control problem than a knife wound in the arm that has lacerated only muscle tissue. Such a wound in the body can cause massive internal hemorrhage which may not be immediately visible, and thus the first aider might underestimate the seriousness of the injury. In the case of an arm injury, however, the hemorrhage is readily visible, so the natural reaction is to assume that this is the more serious of the two injuries when actually it may not be. The problem of internal hemorrhage is compounded by the fact that not only is it difficult to detect, but there is little the first aider can do to control it. External bleeding, on the other hand, can be controlled by the first aider with the use of various pressure techniques, thus helping to reduce its possible life-threatening nature.

CIRCULATION OF BLOOD

Blood is the life-giving substance which is constantly being pumped throughout our bodies by means of the circulatory system. It travels through blood vessels carrying nutrients and oxygen to and removing waste products from each of our body cells. It is important to have some concept of how the circulatory system functions in order to comprehend proper hemorrhage management.

Oxygenated blood is pumped from the lungs to the various parts of the body through blood vessels called arteries. Arteries branch into arterioles and eventually into the smallest blood vessels called capillaries. Capillaries are the vessels which come into direct contact with the individual cells of the body. It is at this level that the exchange process occurs between oxygen, nutrients, and waste products. From the capillaries blood flows into venules, then into the large vessels called veins, which transport the blood back to the heart where the cycle continues.*

CLASSIFICATION OF HEMORRHAGE

Hemorrhage is the condition whereby blood escapes from the blood vessels. It may occur as a result of disease or trauma to these vessels. Generally, it is not necessary to know what type of hemorrhage is occurring in order to control it properly; however, recognition will assist the first aider in evaluating the seriousness of the hemorrhage. Hemorrhage is classified into three types: *arterial*—bleeding from the arteries; *venous*—bleeding from the veins; and *capillary*—bleeding from the capillaries. Hemorrhage may also be classified as internal or external. Internal bleeding, for example, a perforated ulcer, is harder to recognize because it is not readily visible. External hemorrhage is quite evident, as the blood can be seen flowing from the wound.

EXTERNAL HEMORRHAGE

It is important for the first aider to be able to recognize whether the bleeding he observes may be coming from an artery, vein, or capillary.

Arterial, Venous, or Capillary Hemorrhage

Blood traveling through the arteries comes directly from the heart and is bright red in color because it has been freshly oxygenated. In

---

*For a diagram of the blood transfer system, see Appendix C.

arterial hemorrhage the blood spurts from the wound with each heart beat, and bleeding may be profuse due to the continuous force of the heart's pumping action. Arteries, however, are well protected within body tissue, and are therefore not frequently subject to injury.

Bleeding from veins is usually slow and even. Venous blood, which is returning to the heart, is dark red because it is carrying the wastes of metabolism. A danger associated with venous hemorrhage is the possibility of air being sucked into the vein (air embolism), which could affect the heart's pumping action. Since veins are located fairly close to the skin surface they are more susceptible to injury than arteries.

Capillary hemorrhage, coming from smaller vessels, appears as a steady oozing of blood.

Of the three types of hemorrhage, arterial hemorrhage is considered the most serious because it is the most difficult to control. It is possible for an individual to exsanguinate (lose all his blood) from venous bleeding, although this type of hemorrhage is usually more controllable. Any one of the three types of hemorrhage can occur either externally or internally.

The average adult has five to six quarts of blood in his circulatory system. An adult may lose up to a pint of blood with little or no serious effect. However, the loss of one quart is considered serious. It is important that the first aider know how to control hemorrhage quickly and effectively in order to prevent an individual from going into shock or exsanguinating.

First Aid Procedures for External Hemorrhage

Minor hemorrhage may be controlled simply by elevating the injured portion of the body. This method is usually effective only with minor wounds such as small lacerations to the hands or feet. For example, in the case of a lacerated finger, the individual may control bleeding simply by holding the injured hand in the air for a few minutes. Similarly, if an individual is bleeding from a foot or ankle injury, he should be made to lie down, with the injured leg elevated.

Often applications of ice or cold water will assist in the control of hemorrhage. Simply apply a sterile dressing over the wound and a cold pack directly over the dressing. Cold applications are especially effective in preventing swelling. They also help to control superficial internal hemorrhage, as described under Contusions in Chapter 4.

Major hemorrhages require more elaborate control procedures. In the order of severity of bleeding the methods used are: (1) direct pressure, (2) indirect pressure, and (3) tourniquet, as a last resort.

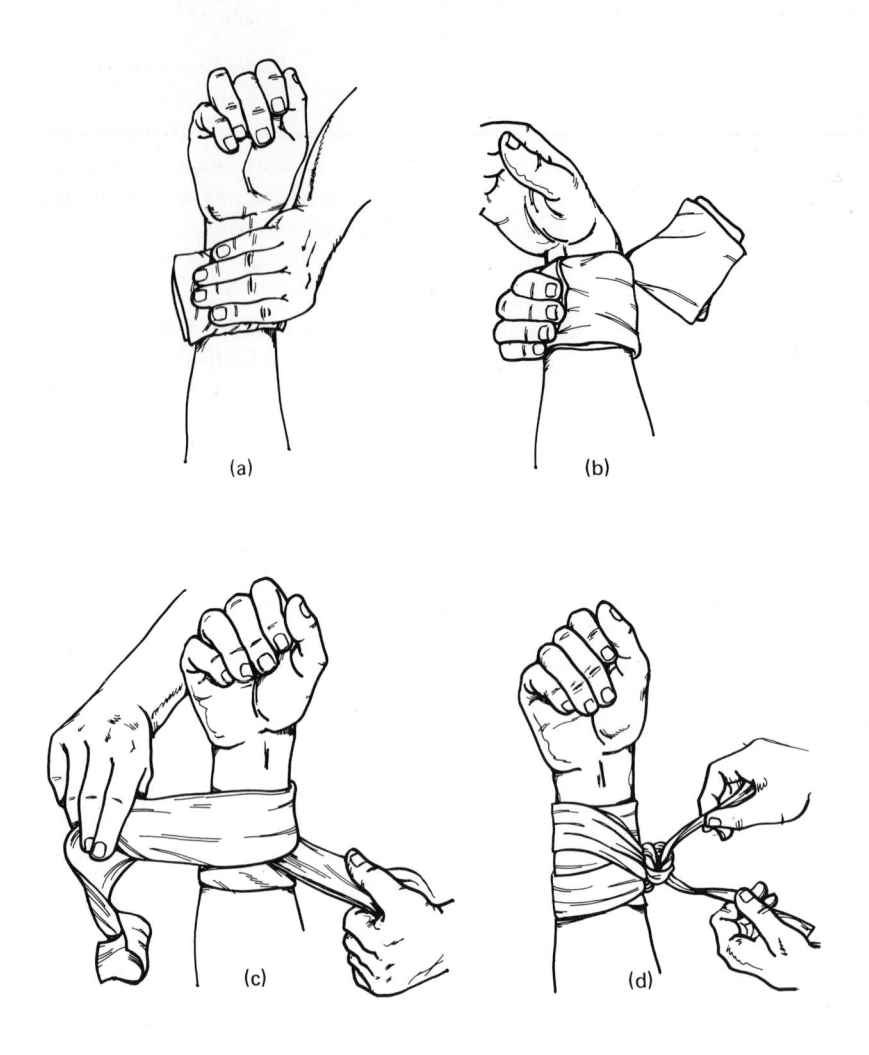

Figure 3.1 To apply a pressure dressing: place a sterile dressing or several layers of dressings over the wound (a) and (b), and snugly secure the dressings in place by a roller bandage or strip of cloth (c) and (d).

Direct Pressure

Perhaps the single most effective method in the control of external hemorrhage is the application of direct pressure over the wound. The first aider should apply sterile gauze pads directly over the wound and then apply a tight roller bandage or cravat to maintain pressure (Figure 3.1). Care should be taken not to wrap the pressure dressing so tightly that circulation is constricted. In areas of the body where pressure dressings can not be easily applied (wound to the face, neck, and certain areas of the head), the sterile dressing can be held in place with adhesive tape. When first aid supplies are not available, items such as clean towels, wash cloths, handkerchiefs, and so on, may be used as a dressing. If the first aider finds himself in a situation where even these items are not available, he may apply direct pressure simply by placing his hand tightly over the wound until the bleeding subsides. Figure 3.2 shows the proper position for the hands in applying direct pressure. Once a direct pressure dressing has been applied, pressure should not be released until the first aider is sure the bleeding has completely stopped or the individual has been taken to a medical facility. Coagulated blood at the wound site should not be tampered with as hemorrhage may reoccur. Clotting is the blood's natural mechanism to control hemorrhage, but it does not occur instantaneously. It may take as long as three to ten minutes for a clot to develop, therefore it is imperative that direct pressure be maintained for at least this period of time. In cases of severe bleeding, especially arterial hemorrhage, clotting may not occur and additional first aid procedures must be used to bring the hemorrhage under control.

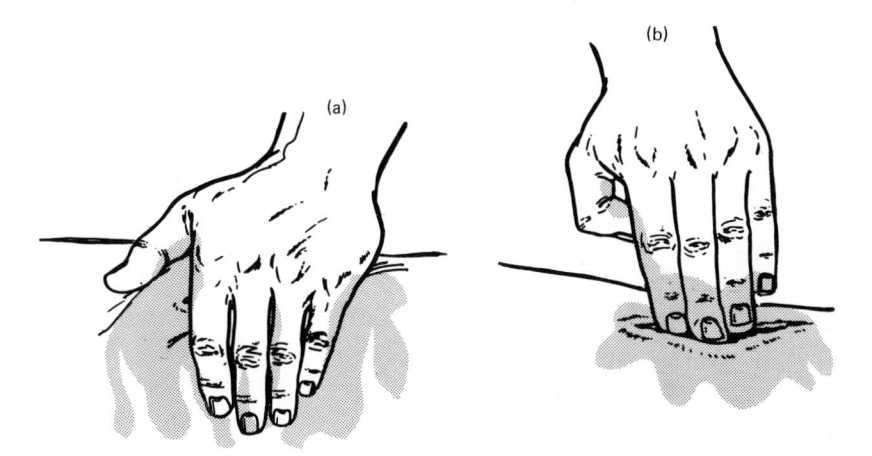

Figure 3.2 Direct pressure hemorrhage control is achieved by: (a) applying pressure directly to the wound site, using a sterile dressing or the hand; (b) inserting the fingers directly into the wound to compress the injured vessels.

Indirect Pressure (Pressure Points)

If hemorrhage is so severe that the direct pressure method is ineffective, indirect pressure (often called *pressure point* control) may be used in addition. This method consists of applying pressure to the artery supplying the injury site. There are 22 points in the body (11 on each side)

[50] Hemorrhage Control

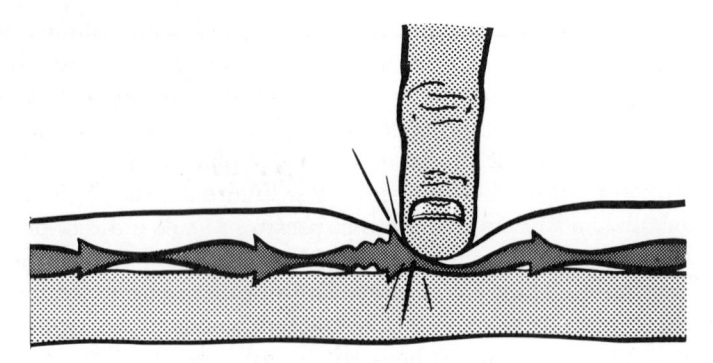

Figure 3.3 Mechanism of indirect pressure hemorrhage control.

where an artery can be compressed or "pinched" against a bone to control and check the flow of blood beyond this point (Figure 3.3).

The six major pressure points (Figure 3.4) are:

1. *Temporal* (side of the head in front of ear): for control of scalp bleeding.
2. *Facial* (along jaw, midway between chin and ear): for control of bleeding in the cheek.
3. *Carotid* (side of neck below jaw): for control of head and neck bleeding.
4. *Subclavian* (between clavicle and first rib): for control of bleeding in armpit, shoulder, and upper chest.
5. *Brachial* (middle portion of upper arm): for control of arm bleeding.
6. *Femoral* (groin area, between hip and pubis): for control of leg bleeding.

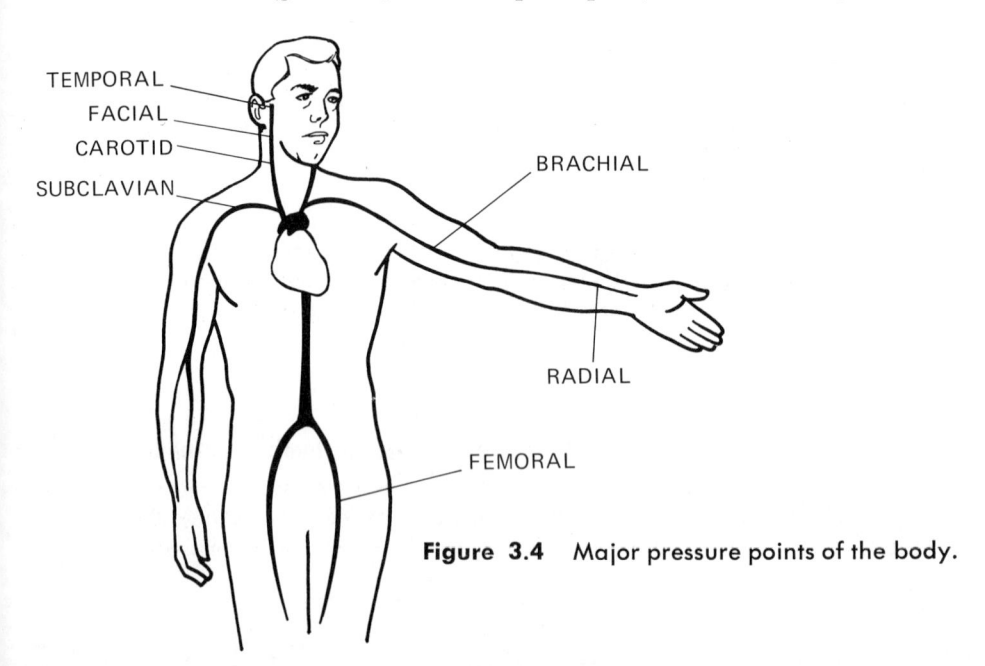

Figure 3.4 Major pressure points of the body.

Hemorrhage Control   [51]

Pressure applied to the brachial and femoral arteries at the proper point is effective in controlling hemorrhage in the extremities. Figure 3.5 illustrates the correct position of the hands for applying femoral and brachial pressure. In all cases it is important to apply sufficient pressure to check the bleeding, and to maintain this pressure continuously until medical attention is reached.

A combination of a pressure dressing at the wound site and indirect pressure at the supplying artery should succeed in controlling even the most severe hemorrhage, provided that the pressure is held long enough to allow the clotting mechanism to function. If pressure is released too soon, clots which have begun to form will be forced loose by the pressure of the blood, and hemorrhage will resume.

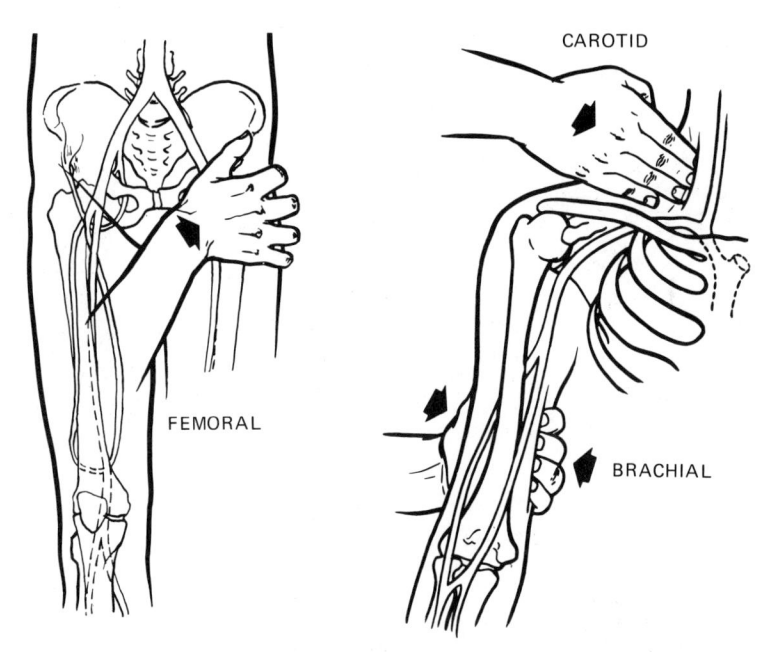

Figure 3.5 Proper hand position for applying femoral and brachial pressure.

Tourniquet

In instances where hemorrhage is so severe (for example, torn or partially amputated limbs) that the methods of hemorrhage control discussed above fail to control the bleeding, a tourniquet may be used, but only as a last resort, that is, when a life is in jeopardy. The reason is that when a tourniquet is applied properly, the blood supply is com-

[52] Hemorrhage Control

pletely cut off to all points below the tourniquet. Tourniquets left on for an extended period of time cause tissue death (gangrene), and the part may have to be amputated. In addition, the pressure from the tourniquet may cause damage to surrounding nerves and blood vessels. Thus a tourniquet should be used only as a last measure after all other methods of hemorrhage control have proven ineffective.

If it becomes necessary to use a tourniquet, proceed as follows:

1. There are several commercially made tourniquets available to the first aider, and if at all possible one of these should be used as they are designed specifically for this purpose. If a commercial tourniquet is not available, a triangular bandage folded several times so that it is at least two inches wide and three or four layers thick, a towel or handkerchief similarly folded, a necktie, or a length of rubber tubing may be used. Never use items such as string or wire as they tend to cut into the skin and cause damage to the underlying tissue and nerves.

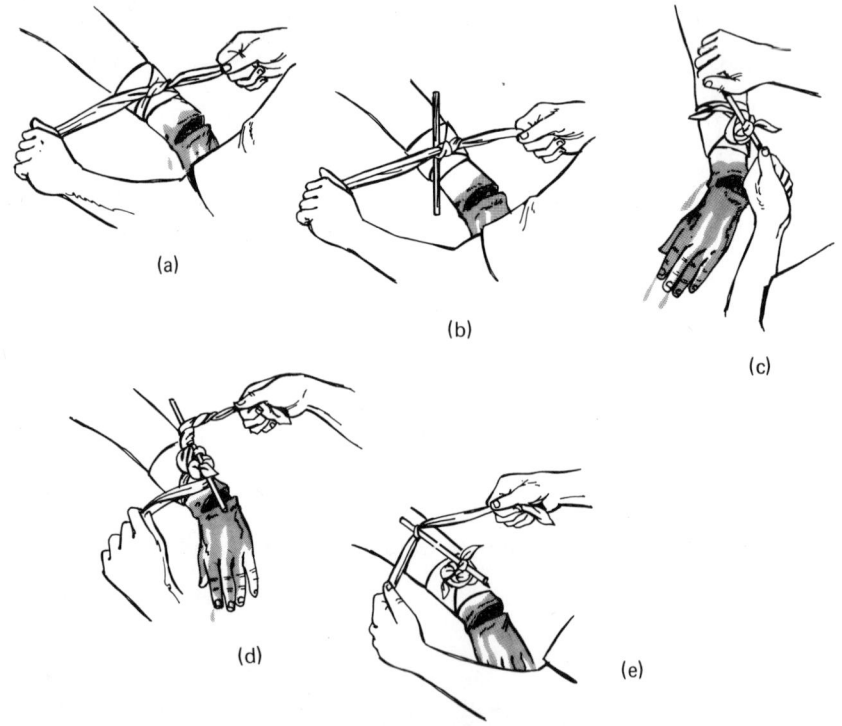

Figure 3.6 To apply a tourniquet properly: (a) place a 2-inch bandage as close to edge of wound as possible and secure with single knot; (b) place a stick or similar object in knot and secure; (c) twist knotted stick until hemorrhage ceases; (d) and (e) secure in place.

2. Position the tourniquet above and as close to the edges of the wound as possible. The tourniquet must be placed between the wound and the heart in order to be effective.
3. The tourniquet may then be applied as shown in Figure 3.6.
4. The tourniquet should be tightened only enough to control the immediate bleeding. Once this has been done, do not continue to tighten the tourniquet. There are many theories as to whether a tourniquet should be loosened from time to time. It is generally best never to loosen the tourniquet until medical help is reached. Loosening the tourniquet may result in uncontrolled hemorrhage and circulation of blood clots and toxins from the damaged tissue.
5. Immediately after applying the tourniquet, note the time. This is important so that medical personnel will know how long the circulation has been constricted. A large "TK" should be written on the injured individual's forehead so that medical personnel will immediately recognize the life-threatening nature of the individual's injuries.

AMPUTATIONS

If an extremity of the body (such as a finger, toe, arm, or leg) has been completely amputated, bleeding can best be controlled by a combination of direct and indirect pressure. Bleeding in such cases is usually less severe than one night expect, since the injured blood vessels tend to constrict due to their natural elasticity. In view of recent advances in restorative surgery, the amputated portion should be retained and transported to the hospital with the injured individual. If possible, wrap the amputated portion in a cold wet dressing.

NOSE BLEEDS

Simple nose bleeds usually last for only a few minutes and are easy to control. Generally, the individual should be made to sit down and remain quiet. The head should be slightly elevated, but not to the extent that blood will interfere with the airway. Direct pressure may be applied by pinching the nostrils together (Figure 3.7). An alternate method is to roll a sterile dressing and place it between the individual's gum and upper lip. Pressure must be continuously applied for at least 6 to 8 minutes. Often the application of ice packs or cold water on the forehead immediately above the nose or across the bridge of the nose may help control the bleeding. If hemorrhage persists more than 10 to 15 minutes, the individual should be taken to a medical facility for professional assistance.

[54] Hemorrhage Control

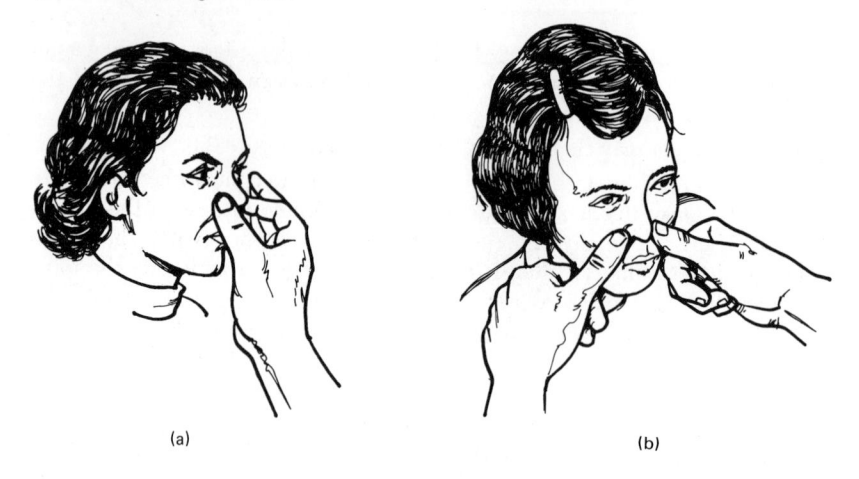

(a) (b)

Figure 3.7 A nosebleed may be controlled (a) by pinching the nostrils directly, or (b) by applying pressure with the thumbs to the supply arteries below the nose.

INTERNAL HEMORRHAGE

In most instances, internal hemorrhage will not be visible to the first aider because the blood will be escaping into the internal cavities of the body. Internal hemorrhage can be profuse and life-threatening, as there may be trauma to large blood vessels and vital organs. This type of hemorrhage usually occurs as a result of a crushing or blunt injury to the body. It may also occur as a result of disease or illness, as in the case of a perforated ulcer. Minor internal bleeding may also occur in the form of a contusion, a soft tissue injury discussed in Chapter 4.

Indicators of Internal Hemorrhage

Generally, the indicators of internal bleeding are the same as those for shock (described fully in Chapter 5). More definitive signs may, however, be evident. These include vomiting or coughing up red or dark clotted blood, and hemorrhage from any of the body openings such as the mouth, ears, nose, etc. Internal hemorrhage should always be suspected in cases of closed fractures. The accumulation of large amounts of blood in the fracture area is evident through severe swelling.

First Aid Procedures for Internal Hemorrhage

The first aider can do little to control internal hemorrhage, but there are specific procedures he can follow to prevent the injured individual from going into shock. The most dangerous forms of internal bleeding are those which have occurred as a result of crushing injuries and where large amounts of blood are escaping into the chest or abdominal cavities. These victims are in extreme danger and should be transported to a medical facility immediately. Until professional help takes over, the injured should be treated in the same manner as an individual who is in shock. It is most important that these individuals be given nothing by mouth as they often will need to undergo surgery to control the hemorrhage.

{ 4 }

SOFT TISSUE INJURIES

A soft tissue injury or wound may be defined as any break in the skin or mucous membrane which interrupts the continuity of the skin or membrane. Such injuries, whether external or internal, may vary in severity from a mere pinprick to a mutilation serious enough to require amputation. The severity depends on the area of the body involved and the force with which the injury was sustained.

Wounds are classified as open or closed. Closed wounds such as *contusions* (bruises) or *hematoma* (blood clots) may at first appear minor, but may be a sign of a more serious internal injury. Open wounds are visible since blood and other body fluids are seen to escape. In addition to blood loss and its relationship to shock, open wounds are susceptible to contamination, which leads to infection.

CLOSED WOUNDS

Injuries sustained from a blow with a blunt object result in contusions, or bruises. The skin is not penetrated, but the blow ruptures blood vessels internally and hemorrhage occurs (Figure 4.1). When deeper blood vessels are injured, hematoma may form. If the blow is severe enough, in addition to the crushed tissue, internal organs may rupture or bones may fracture. Contusions should not be taken lightly as they may be the only outward sign of these more serious internal injuries.

[58] Soft Tissue Injuries

— CRUSHED TISSUE

— BLOOD CLOT FORMATION

— BLOOD SEEPAGE INTO SURROUNDING TISSUE

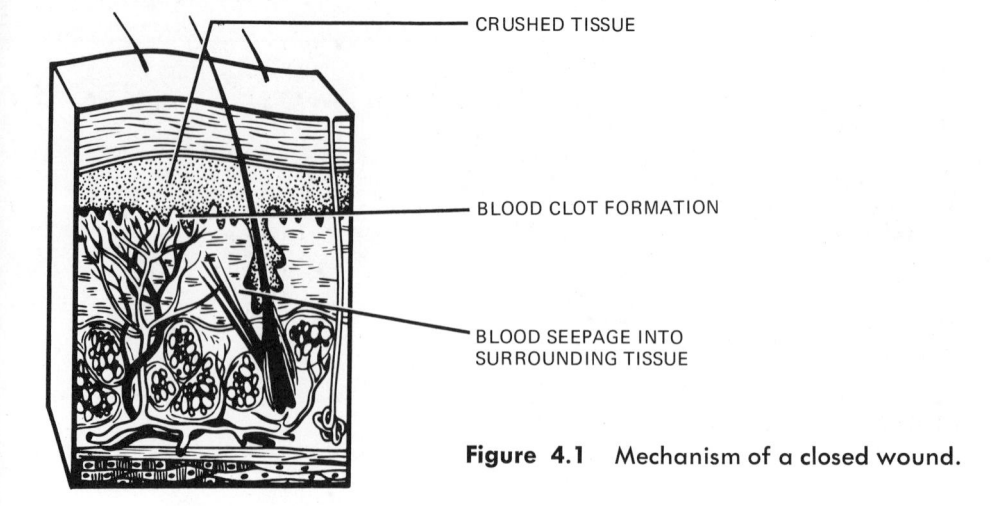

Figure 4.1   Mechanism of a closed wound.

Indicators of Contusions

In contusions the site of injury may become red and tender to the touch, and swelling often occurs. Blood seeping into the tissues causes the skin to discolor or form a black-and-blue mark.

First Aid Procedures for Closed Wounds

If the bruise site is small, no real medical attention is required. Nevertheless cold applications may be applied at the time of injury to control the hemorrhage, and a small pressure dressing may also be applied. However, if the bruise does not seem to heal or the blow was severe, as from a blunt object, medical attention should be sought.

OPEN WOUNDS

Injuries sustained from a blow with a sharp object cause the skin to be torn open. Open wounds vary in severity and type according to the object inflicting the injury. An ice pick makes a puncture hole; a shattered windshield can leave a jagged tear. Open wounds are generally classified as abrasions, punctures, incisions, or lacerations. Additionally, tissue may be avulsed, crushed, or amputated (Figure 4.2).

Abrasions occur as a result of a scraping or rubbing action. Most abrasions only involve the outer layer of skin, with minor bleeding. The most serious consequence to be considered is contamination, as dirt and bacteria may be ground into the skin in the scraping or rubbing action. An example of an abrasion is a skinned knee.

(a) PUNCTURE

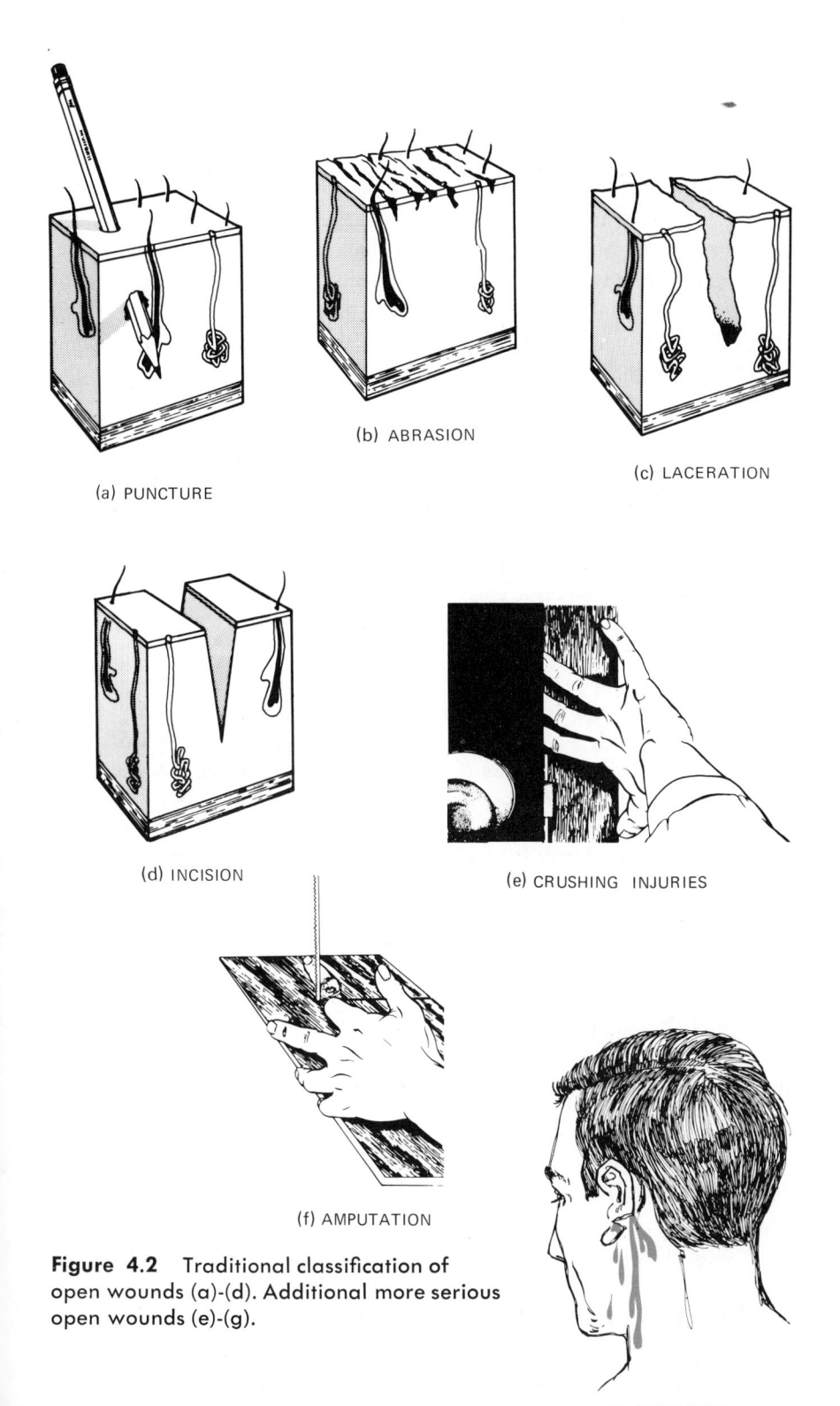

(b) ABRASION

(c) LACERATION

(d) INCISION

(e) CRUSHING INJURIES

(f) AMPUTATION

(g) AVULSION

Figure 4.2 Traditional classification of open wounds (a)-(d). Additional more serious open wounds (e)-(g).

Punctures are the result of a stabbing by a sharp pointed object such as a nail or an ice pick, inflicting a hole of varying size. The object may merely penetrate the surface, as in the case of splinters, or it can become embedded deep in muscle or organ tissue. Puncture wounds generally do not bleed freely, but are susceptible to contamination and run the risk of causing severe destruction of underlying tissue.

Incisions result from contact with sharp smooth-edged objects. They may penetrate all layers of the skin and bleed quite freely. An example of an incision would be a razor or knife cut.

Lacerations, perhaps the most common types of open wounds, result from the tearing of tissue leaving a jagged-edged injury. Such injuries may bleed freely and are susceptible to contamination. Considerable underlying tissue destruction may occur concurrently. Typical examples of lacerations are those occurring from contact with broken glass and protruding metal.

In addition to these four traditional types of open wounds, three others may be described: avulsion, crushing, and traumatic amputation. These are serious open injuries often associated with motor vehicle and industrial accidents.

In an *avulsion* a piece of the soft tissue is torn loose or left hanging as a flap. The wound may or may not bleed, depending on what caused the avulsion. With severe injuries, contamination and interruption to nerve and blood supplies may cause serious complications. Common examples of avulsions are earring injuries to the ear lobe.

A *crushing* injury occurs when a part of the body—often a hand or arm—is caught by or run through a piece of machinery. This is a serious injury with possible open fractures and surface lacerations. Bleeding may be slight as the vessels are crushed to the point of closure. However, the greatest damage is to the underlying tissues, which are literally crushed.

Traumatic *amputations* may occur from extreme tearing action to a limb of the body. Jagged skin and bone edges are apparent; there may or may not be extensive bleeding. The amputated portion should be located and transported to the medical facility for possible reattachment to the victim.

Major Hemorrhaging Wounds

If the wound is hemorrhaging the prime responsibility of the first aider is to control that hemorrhage, using one or a combination of the techniques discussed in Chapter 3, namely, elevation, direct pressure, indirect pressure, and as a final resort, tourniquet. In addition, every precaution should be taken to prevent contamination. This can be accomplished simply by covering the wound site with a sterile dressing or a clean piece of cloth. Once the hemorrhage is controlled and a pressure dressing applied, immediately transport the individual to a medical facility.

Minor Hemorrhaging Wounds

Minor open wounds do not always require medical attention. Usually the bleeding can be controlled by elevation and direct pressure. The chief concern with these wounds is the danger of contamination. To minimize the possibility of contamination, the wound site should be cleansed thoroughly. Plain soap and water have proven best for this purpose. If necessary the area may be soaked in soapy water for about 15 minutes. Any imbedded foreign objects, such as gravel, stones, or pieces of asphalt, which do not wash out by themselves in the bleeding or soaking action should not be removed by the first aider but should be left to a professional for their removal. Indiscriminate removal may initiate severe bleeding. Antiseptics should not be used except under the direction of a physician, as they may destroy tissue or mask the developing signs of infection. After the area has been cleansed thoroughly, a dressing and bandage may be applied. The wound site should be observed for signs of infection (discussed below) and if it develops, medical attention should be sought.

INFECTION

Since disease-producing (pathogenic) micro-organisms are present everywhere, any wound can become infected. Most susceptible to infection are wounds which do not bleed freely, wounds in which torn tissue or skin falls back into place preventing the entrance of air (particularly true of puncture wounds), and wounds which involve crushing of the tissues. The most common pathogenic organisms affecting man include the streptococci and staphlococci, colon bacillus, tetanus bacillus, and gas bacillus. Tetanus and gas bacillus are common in puncture wounds because they grow in the absence of oxygen. However, for gas gangrene to develop, massive destruction and death of tissues seem to be necessary.

Indicators of Infection

Signs of infection include redness, heat, pain, swelling, pus, and throbbing at the wound site. It may take anywhere from six hours to four days for all these signs to develop. If in addition red streaks are seen to radiate from the wound site, this is a sign that the infection is spreading,

[62]   Soft Tissue Injuries

and immediate medical attention should be sought. When indicators of infection appear, the first aider should not attempt to handle this emergency. Elaborate medical techniques are required to diagnose and treat infections, so time should not be lost in trying to handle this situation without professional supervision.

Tetanus

Tetanus (also known as lockjaw) is caused by a rod-shaped bacillus which is widely dispersed in the environment. Its spores and organisms may be found almost everywhere, including on the body. The bacillus grows best in an oxygen-free (anaerobic) atmosphere such as exists in deep puncture wounds, but any open wound which does not bleed freely may breed the tetanus infection. Tetanus is entirely preventable through immunization. Two types of immunization widely used in the prevention and treatment of tetanus are (1) toxoid vaccine, which is active immunization and gives protection for many years, and (2) antitoxin, which is passive immunization and short-lived. If an individual is exposed to possible tetanus bacillus and has previously had the toxoid, a booster shot may be given to restimulate production of antibodies; this gives almost

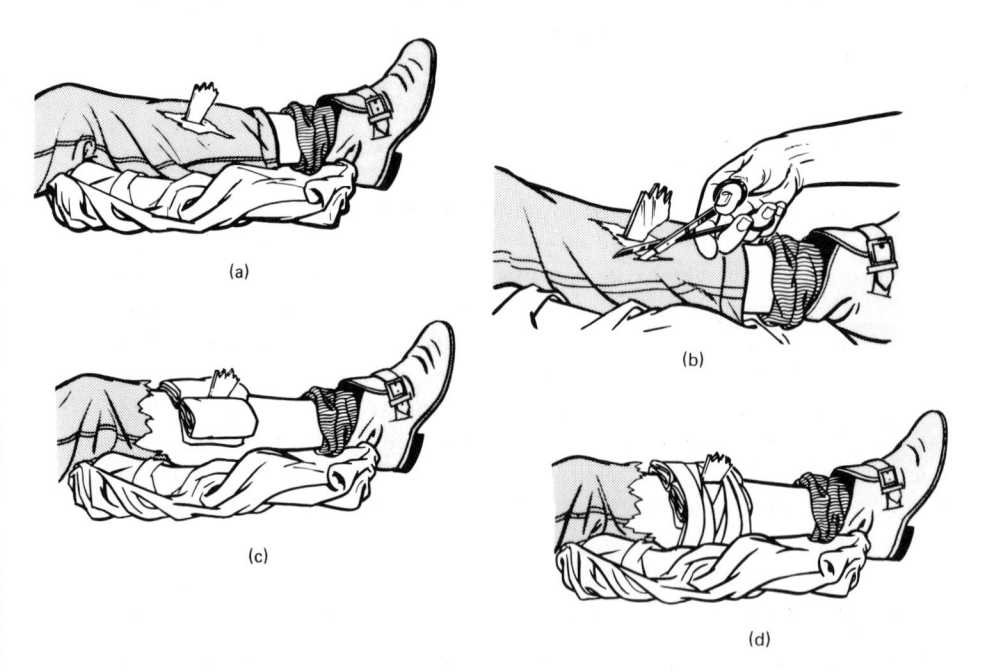

Figure 4.3   In stabilizing an embedded object the first aider should (a) never remove or move the object; (b) carefully cut clothing away from around the wound site; (c) stabilize with bulky dressings; and (d) secure with bandages, avoiding covering the object.

certain protection against the onset of infection. However, if the individual has never had the active toxoid, tetanus antitoxin may be administered. This consists of an injection of the antibodies necessary to control the tetanus bacillus. The shot is effective only for the current injury; subsequent injections of the antitoxin may produce sensitization and a severe reaction. Although tetanus remains a dangerous infection, it can be controlled through the administration of either toxoid or antitoxin; hence the number of cases of lockjaw which develop annually are relatively few.

Lockjaw develops from four days to three weeks after the bacteria enter the body. Early symptoms are stiffness of the neck muscles and painful spasms of the jaw muscles. As the disease progresses, the jaws may "lock" and the individual assumes a peculiar facial expression—raised eyebrows with droopy facial muscles around the mouth. Convulsions, high fever, and respiratory distress may also follow. Medical treatment is complicated and may require months of hospitalization and hyperbaric chamber treatments.

SPECIAL WOUNDS

Embedded Objects

When a foreign body remains lodged in the soft tissues, it is known as an embedded object. Almost anything can become embedded—pieces of glass, metal, pebbles, or fishhooks. The first aider should not attempt to remove an embedded object as this may cause severe hemorrhage due to the releasing of the pressure on the severed blood vessels. Removal of the object may also cause further injury to the surrounding muscles and tissues. An exception is made for removing an embedded object if it occurs in the cheek. Because the tissue in this area is relatively thin and retention of the object causes hemorrhage within the mouth as well as externally, removal of the object is necessary in order to maintain a clear airway. But removal should be attempted by the first aider only if the object will slide out easily from the direction of entry. If resistance is met, the object should be left in place for surgical removal.

First Aid Procedures for Embedded Objects

The first aider must control what external bleeding is occurring, either by direct pressure at the edges of the wound or through pressure at the supplying artery (indirect pressure). Hemorrhage may be slight, however, as the embedded object is supplying the pressure internally. A bulky dressing should be applied (Figure 4.3) to stabilize the object and prevent its moving during transport to a medical facility. In addition the area should be immobilized in the same manner as a fracture, in order to further prevent movement.

Gunshot Wounds

The type of wound inflicted by a bullet will depend upon the weapon and the ammunition used. The injury may appear quite slight, as in small caliber weapons, or it may be massive, as with a close-range shotgun. Much of the damage inflicted is to the internal organs, which produces massive internal hemorrhage. Often there are two wound sites—at the points of entry and exit of the bullet. It is important that the victim be checked for two wounds, because the exit wound may be huge but the entry wound merely a small puncture.

First Aid Procedures for Gunshot Wounds

The first aider should treat the indicators present. If massive hemorrhage is occurring, direct or indirect pressure must be applied along with the proper dressing. If it appears that the bone has been fractured, immobilization will also be necessary. Shock, often due to internal hemorrhage, must be suspected and cared for in all instances. All gunshot wounds must be reported to legal authorities. The first aider should be mindful of this and do nothing that might destroy helpful evidence concerning the incident, whether it be an accident, suicide, homicide, or an attempt at such.

Open Chest Wounds

When the chest cavity is penetrated by a sharp object, bullet, or fractured rib, an injury known as a "sucking chest wound" may result. Air entering and exiting from the site creates the characteristic sucking or hissing sound as the injured individual attempts to breathe. He is unable to fill his lungs with air as in normal respiration. Medically, this type of injury may be termed a *pneumothorax* (presence of air outside the lung but within the chest cavity). In this type of injury, the pleural sac between the ribs and the lung is perforated, and air and/or blood seep into the chest cavity. As a result of the air or blood accumulation, the lung cannot expand normally and the lung is compressed, causing a loss of function or total collapse (Figure 4.4).

Indicators of Open Chest Wounds

The major indicator of an open chest wound is the hole in the chest or an embedded object protruding from the chest wall. The injured in-

Soft Tissue Injuries [65]

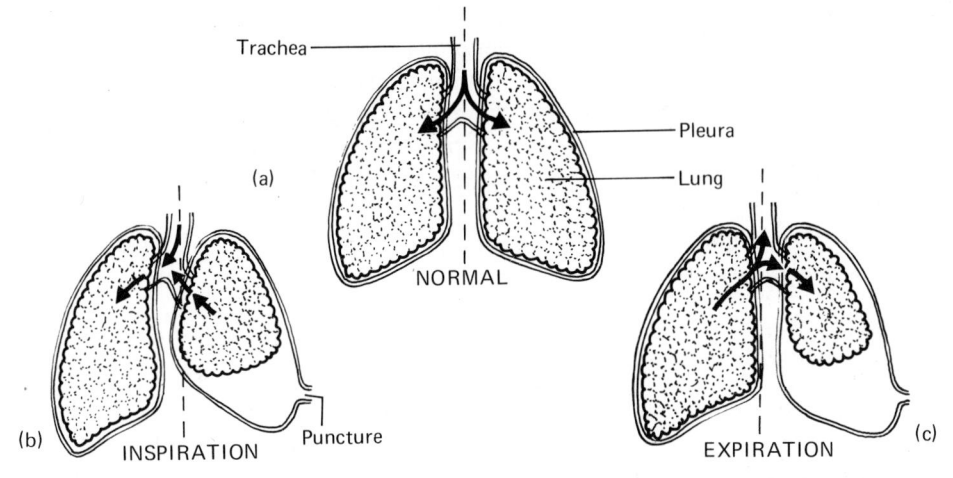

Figure 4.4 In a pneumothorax the normal relationship (a) of the lung and pleural sac is affected. When the pleura is punctured by an object, air is allowed to enter the pleural cavity. As a result the lung collapses and is pushed toward the uninjured side as the individual breathes in (b). During expiration the shift is in the opposite direction (c), which may also affect heart action.

dividual has difficulty breathing, and if the lung has been penetrated, he may be spitting or coughing up bright red, frothy blood. With each breath a sucking or hissing sound will be heard. There may also be signs of shock, especially if hemorrhage is occurring within the chest cavity.

First Aid Procedures for Open Chest Wounds

The most immediate procedure is to seal the external hole and prevent air from continuing to enter the chest cavity. Nothing can be done externally by the first aider to control internal hemorrhage if it is occurring simultaneously. The external hole should be sealed with a nonporous

Figure 4.5 A pneumothorax must be sealed as quickly as possible with a large nonporous dressing. The first aider's hand may be used temporarily.

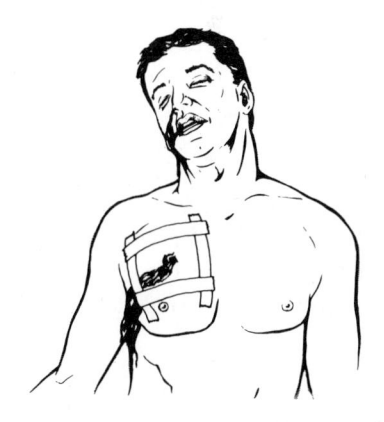

dressing such as aluminum foil, plastic wrap, plastic bags, petrolatum saturated gauze dressing, and nonporous tape (Figure 4.5). If nothing else is available, the first aider's hand may be used as a temporary seal. If the object is still embedded at the injury site, do not attempt to remove it, but seal the wound the best way possible with the object intact. The airway should be cleared and maintained while the victim is given care for shock. If there is no penetrating object the individual may be placed lying on his injured side during transportation to a medical facility, as this will help further seal the opening.

Open Abdominal Wounds

The abdominal region of the body is vulnerable to injury because its only protection is a muscle sheath. Deep injuries to this region may cause hemorrhage to occur internally as a result of trauma to the vital organs and blood vessels located within the cavity. If the mechanism of injury is sharp, the skin and muscle sheath may be torn, leaving the intestines exposed. This type of an injury may be serious, even though the intestines are often surgically repositioned and the individual recovers fully. Complications occur due to the contamination which results when the intestine is ruptured.

Indicators of Open Abdominal Injuries

The most obvious sign of this type of injury is that the intestines are visible and may be protruding from the abdominal cavity. The individual may also be in severe pain, with nausea, vomiting, and spasms of the abdominal muscles; he may also be in severe shock.

First Aid Procedures for Open Abdominal Wounds

Place the injured individual on his back and cover the exposed intestines with a large bulky dressing. Be careful not to handle the intestines, because they rupture easily due to their thin membranes. Since the intestines are normally coiled up in the abdomen, by improper handling several feet may eject instead of the few inches that were originally protruding. The dressing should be moistened with water, preferably sterile, and then secured in place with tape or large triangular bandages. Minimal pressure should be applied during the process of bandaging. Extreme pressure may cause the intestine to rupture. The injured individual should be checked and given care for shock, and transported to a medical facility as soon as possible. Nothing should be administered by mouth, because surgery is the usual definitive care for the injured individual.

Genital Organ Injuries

Injuries to the genital organs usually result from kicks, blows, straddle accidents, impact with blunt instruments, or contact with sharp instruments. In addition to an apparent injury to the genital organs, damage may also have occurred to the urethra, bladder, intestine, and internal reproductive organs.

Indicators of Genital Injury

Injuries of the genital organs are usually accompanied by severe pain, swelling, and hemorrhage. Avulsions may occur or objects may be found inserted or embedded in the organs.

First Aid Procedures for Genital Injury

Any embedded or inserted object must be left as found and stabilized to prevent further injury. Hemorrhage can be controlled with direct pressure in the form of a diaper-style pressure dressing. The injured individual should be lying down with the hips and legs elevated if possible. Check and give care for shock, and retain any avulsed tissue for reattachment or grafting. The injured individual should be transported to a medical facility without delay, preferably via ambulance.

Eye Injuries

The eye is probably the most important sense organ and any injury or interference that affects the eyes should be handled with the greatest care. Proper initial care not only helps to relieve pain but also helps prevent permanent damage and loss of vision. Whenever a first aider must examine the eye or care for eye injuries, he should attempt to do so with clean hands, as the eye is sensitive and one must be very gentle not to aggravate any existing injuries. Eye injuries may be classified in three categories: (1) foreign objects, (2) lacerations and contusions, and (3) chemical and heat burns.

First Aid Procedures for Eye Injuries

Probably the most common eye injury results when foreign objects such as dirt, dust, or insects become lodged on the outer surface of the eyeball or under the eyelid. Although not serious, this type of injury may be very incapacitating. Most of these foreign objects are removed by the mechanism of the body's own tears. Simply pulling the upper lid over the lower lid will aid in this tearing action. If the tears do not wash out

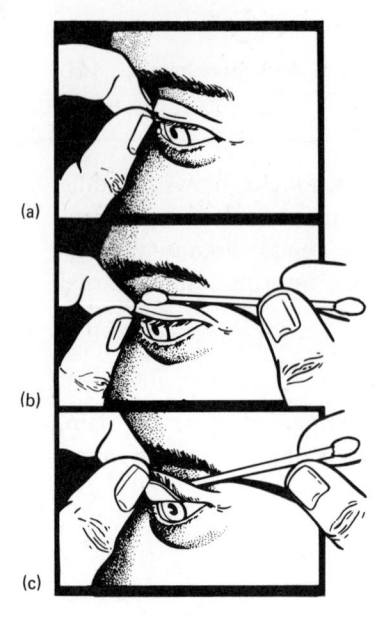

Figure 4.6 When removing a foreign object from the upper eyelid the first aider should (a) grasp the upper lid between thumb and forefinger; (b) fold lid over a cotton swab or similar rounded tip; while (c) the individual looks downward exposing the upper surface of the eyeball.

the object, the first aider may attempt its removal in either of the following ways:

Upper lid. Grasp the upper eyelid with the thumb and forefinger. Fold the lid upward over a rounded object such as a swab, while the individual looks downward. This exposes the surface of the upper lid and globe of the eye. The first aider may continue by rinsing the exposed area with water, or if the object is visible, remove the object with a corner of a clean cloth or swab (Figure 4.6). (No dry cotton should be used around the eye.)

Lower lid. Grasp the lower lid with the thumb and forefinger and pull down the lower lid while the individual looks upward. The exposed area

Figure 4.7 Dressing and stabilization of an embedded object in or near the eye.

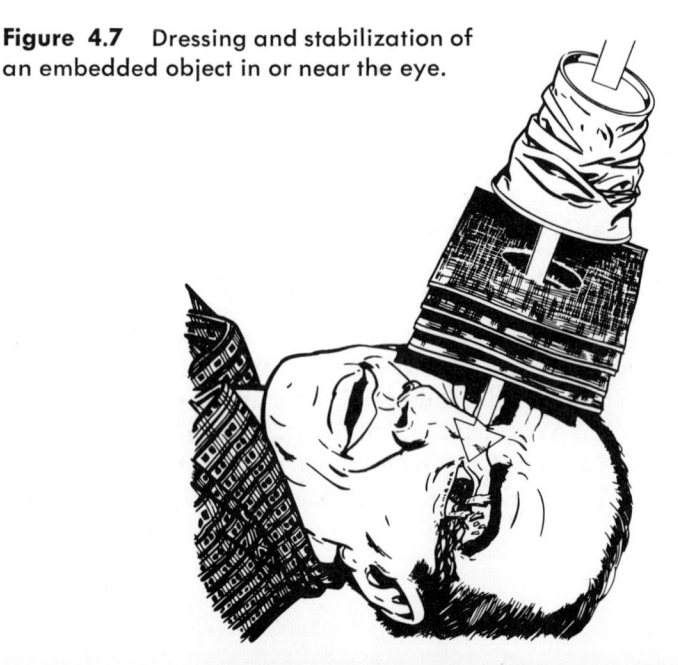

may now be rinsed with water, or if the object is visible, it may be removed in the same manner as for the upper lid.

If the foreign object is not easily removable by the above-described procedures, the eyes should be covered (both eyes as the eyes work together) with a soft loose dressing, and the individual taken to a medical facility for proper removal of the object. If large objects are embedded in the eyeball itself, or in the surrounding soft tissue, no attempt should be made by the first aider to remove the object. The embedded object should be stabilized and protected as previously described for embedded objects (Figure 4.7). These are serious injuries, which may result in loss of sight. Reassurance and comfort are important aspects of the total care given to an individual with a serious eye injury.

Lacerations and contusions may also occur to the soft tissue surrounding the eye or to the eyeball itself. These injuries may appear far more serious than they really are. If the eyelid is lacerated but the globe of the eye is untouched, the individual's sight is usually not affected. However, if the eyeball is lacerated, especially if the jelly-like vitreous fluid is allowed to escape, vision is lost. Hemorrhage from lacerated eyelids may be effectively controlled with direct pressure or pressure dressings. But if the eyeball itself is lacerated, no pressure should be applied. Soft loose dressings may be applied, which will absorb the fluid and aid in the clotting process. Individuals with these types of injuries should be transported to a medical facility as soon as possible.

The third type of injury to the eye is caused by contact with chemicals or heat. Chemical burns are treated by flushing the area with large quantities of water, as discussed under Burns in Chapter 7. An individual receiving burns to the face may suffer damage to the eyelids as will as the eyeball. In such cases it is best that the first aider not attempt to examine the eye; just cover both eyes with soft loose dressings and transport the individual to a medical facility.

Insect Bites

There are a variety of small insects which bite humans. Some individuals are extremely sensitive (anapyhlactic reaction) to the venom injected, especially by bees and wasps. In addition, some insects carry communicable diseases such as malaria and Rocky Mountain fever. The National Safety Council has provided a useful chart identifying nine insects found in the United States and Canada, including chiggers, spiders, bedbugs, mosquitos, bees, and ticks, and giving information on how to protect against and care for the bites of these pests (Figure 4.8).

Figure 4.8 INSECT CHART

	DESCRIPTION	HABITAT	PROBLEM
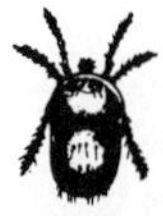 **CHIGGER**	Oval with red velvety covering. Sometimes almost colorless. Larva has six legs. Harmless adult has eight and resembles a small spider. Very tiny—about 1/20-inch long.	Found in low damp places covered with vegetation: shaded woods, high grass or weeds, fruit orchards. Also lawns and golf courses. From Canada to Argentina.	Attaches itself to the skin by inserting mouthparts into a hair follicle. Injects a digestive fluid that causes cells to disintegrate. Then feeds on cell parts. It does not suck blood.
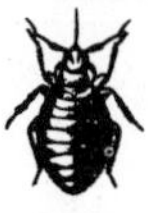 **BEDBUG**	Flat oval body with short broad head and six legs. Adult is reddish brown. Young are yellowish white. Unpleasant pungent odor. From 1/8 to 1/4-inch in length.	Hides in crevices, mattresses, under loose wallpaper during day. At night travels considerable distance to find victims. Widely distributed throughout the world.	Punctures the skin with piercing organs and sucks blood. Local inflammation and welts result from anticoagulant enzyme that bug secretes from salivary glands while feeding.
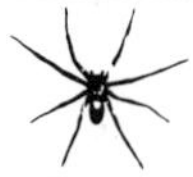 **BROWN RECLUSE SPIDER**	Oval body with eight legs. Light yellow to medium brown. Has distinctive mark shaped like a fiddle on its back. Body from 3/8 to 1/2-inch long, 1/4-inch wide, 3/4-inch from toe-to-toe.	Prefers dark places where it's seldom disturbed. Outdoors: old trash piles, debris and rough ground. Indoors: attics, storerooms, closets. Found in Southern and Midwestern U.S.	Bites producing an almost painless sting that may not be noticed at first. Shy, it bites only when annoyed or surprised. Left alone, it won't bite. Victim rarely sees the spider.
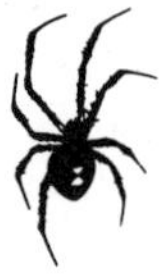 **BLACK WIDOW SPIDER**	Color varies from dark brown to glossy black. Densely covered with short microscopic hairs. Red or yellow hourglass marking on the underside of the female's abdomen. Male does not have this mark and is not poisonous. Overall length with legs extended is 1½ inch. Body is 1/4-inch wide.	Found with eggs and web. Outside: in vacant rodent holes, under stones, logs, in long grass, hollow stumps and brush piles. Inside: in dark corners of barns, garages, piles of stone, wood. Most bites occur in outhouses. Found in Southern Canada, throughout U.S., except Alaska.	Bites causing local redness. Two tiny red spots may appear. Pain follows almost immediately. Larger muscles become rigid. Body temperature rises slightly. Profuse perspiration and tendency toward nausea follow. It's usually difficult to breathe or talk. May cause constipation, urine retention.
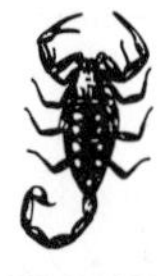 **SCORPION**	Crablike appearance with clawlike pincers. Fleshy postabdomen or "tail" has 5 segments, ending in a bulbous sac and stinger. Two poisonous types: solid straw yellow or yellow with irregular black stripes on back. From 2½ to 4 inches.	Spends days under loose stones, bark, boards, floors of outhouses. Burrows in the sand. Roams freely at night. Crawls under doors into homes. Lethal types are found only in the warm desert-like climate of Arizona and adjacent areas.	Stings by thrusting its tail forward over its head. Swelling or discoloration of the area indicates a non-dangerous, though painful, sting. A dangerously toxic sting doesn't change the appearance of the area, which does become hypersensitive.
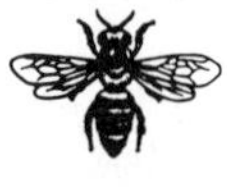 **BEE**	Winged body with yellow and black stripes. Covered with branched or feathery hairs. Makes a buzzing sound. Different species vary from 1/2 to 1 inch in length.	Lives in aerial or underground nests or hives. Widely distributed throughout the world wherever there are flowering plants—from the polar regions to the equator.	Stings with tail when annoyed. Burning and itching with localized swelling occur. Usually leaves venom sac in victim. It takes between 2 and 3 minutes to inject all the venom.
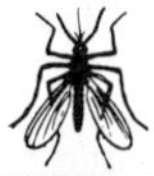 **MOSQUITO**	Small dark fragile body with transparent wings and elongated mouthparts. From 1/8 to 1/4-inch long.	Found in temperate climates throughout the world where the water necessary for breeding is available.	Bites and sucks blood. Itching and localized swelling result. Bite may turn red. Only the female is equipped to bite.
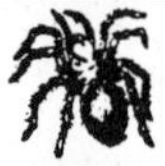 **TARANTULA**	Large dark "spider" with a furry covering. From 6 to 7 inches in toe-to-toe diameter.	Found in Southwestern U.S. and the tropics. Only the tropical varieties are poisonous.	Bites produce pin-prick sensation with negligible effect. It will not bite unless teased.
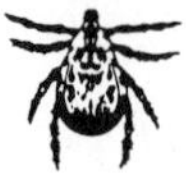 **TICK**	Oval with small head; the body is not divided into definite segments. Grey or brown. Measures from 1/4-inch to 3/4-inch when mature.	Found in all U.S. areas and in parts of Southern Canada, on low shrubs, grass and trees. Carried around by both wild and domestic animals.	Attaches itself to the skin and sucks blood. After removal there is danger of infection, especially if the mouthparts are left in the wound.

Source: Reprinted from *School Safety*, March-April 1971, with permission of the National Safety Council.

SEVERITY	TREATMENT	PROTECTION	
Itching from secreted enzymes results several hours after contact. Small red welts appear. Secondary infection often follows. Degree of irritation varies with individuals.	Lather with soap and rinse several times to remove chiggers. If welts have formed, dab antiseptic on area. Severe lesions may require antihistamine ointment.	Apply proper repellent to clothing, particularly near uncovered areas such as wrists and ankles. Apply to skin. Spray or dust infested areas (lawns, plants) with suitable chemicals.	**CHIGGER**
Affects people differently. Some have marked swelling and considerable irritation while others aren't bothered. Sometimes transmits serious diseases.	Apply antiseptic to prevent possible infection. Bug usually bites sleeping victim, gorges itself completely in 3-5 minutes and departs. It's rarely necessary to remove one.	Spray beds, mattresses, bed springs and baseboards with insecticide. Bugs live in large groups. They migrate to new homes on water pipes and clothing.	**BEDBUG**
In two to eight hours pain may be noticed followed by blisters, swelling, hemorrhage or ulceration. Some people experience rash, nausea, jaundice, chills, fever, cramps or joint pain.	Summon doctor. Bite may require hospitalization for a few days. Full healing may take from 6-8 weeks. Weak adults and children have been known to die.	Use caution when cleaning secluded areas in the home or using machinery usually left idle. Check firewood, inside shoes, packed clothing and bedrolls — frequent hideaways.	**BROWN RECLUSE SPIDER**
Venom is more dangerous than a rattlesnake's but is given in much smaller amounts. About 5 per cent of bite cases result in death. Death is from asphyxiation due to respiratory paralysis. More dangerous for children, to adults its worst feature is pain. Convulsions result in some cases.	Use an antiseptic such as alcohol or hydrogen peroxide on the bitten area to prevent secondary infection. Keep victim quiet and call a doctor. Do not treat as you would a snakebite since this will only increase the pain and chance of infection; bleeding will not remove the venom.	Wear gloves when working in areas where there might be spiders. Destroy any egg sacs you find. Spray insecticide in any area where spiders are usually found, especially under privy seats. Check them out regularly. General cleanliness, paint and light discourage spiders.	**BLACK WIDOW SPIDER**
Excessive salivation and facial contortions may follow. Temperature rises to over 104°. Tongue becomes sluggish. Convulsions, in waves of increasing intensity, may lead to death from nervous exhaustion. First 3 hours most critical.	Apply tourniquet. Keep victim quiet and call a doctor immediately. Do not cut the skin or give pain killers. They increase the killing power of the venom. Antitoxin, readily available to doctors, has proved to be very effective.	Apply a petroleum distillate to any dwelling places that cannot be destroyed. Cats are considered effective predators as are ducks and chickens, though the latter are more likely to be stung and killed. Don't go barefoot at night.	**SCORPION**
If a person is allergic, more serious reactions occur— nausea, shock, unconsciousness. Swelling may occur in another part of the body. Death may result.	Gently scrape (don't pluck) the stinger so venom sac won't be squeezed. Wash with soap and antiseptic. If swelling occurs, contact doctor. Keep victim warm while resting.	Have exterminator destroy nests and hives. Avoid wearing sweet fragrances and bright clothing. Keep food covered. Move slowly or stand still in the vicinity of bees.	**BEE**
Sometimes transmits yellow fever, malaria, encephalitis and other diseases. Scratching can cause secondary infections.	Don't scratch. Lather with soap and rinse to avoid infection. Apply antiseptic to relieve itching.	Destroy available breeding water to check multiplication. Place nets on windows and beds. Use proper repellent.	**MOSQUITO**
Usually no more dangerous than a pin prick. Has only local effects.	Wash and apply antiseptic to prevent the possibility of secondary infection.	Harmless to man, the tarantula is beneficial since it destroys harmful insects.	**TARANTULA**
Sometimes carries and spreads Rocky Mountain spotted fever, tularemia, Colorado tick fever. In a few rare cases, causes paralysis until removed.	Apply heated needle to tick. Gently remove with tweezers so none of the mouthparts are left in skin. Wash with soap and water; apply antiseptic.	Cover exposed parts of body when in tick-infested areas. Use proper repellent. Remove ticks attached to clothes, body. Check neck and hair. Bathe.	**TICK**

Soft Tissue Injuries

Snakebites

The four types of poisonous snakes found in the United States are rattlesnakes, water moccasins, copperheads, and coral snakes (Figure 4.9). The first three are known as "pit vipers" because of the small, deep pits located between the nostrils and eyes on each side of the head. Pit vipers inject venom through long fangs located in their upper jaw, the injected venom acting as a circulatory poison to the victim. Coral snakes, on the other hand, are characterized by their bands of red, black, and yellow. Coral snakes do not have fangs, rather they bite and hang on, injecting venom through a chewing motion. The venom of the coral snake acts on the nervous system of the victim, and is much faster-acting than the venom of the pit viper. Although snakebite death is rare, such injuries can give a great deal of pain and discomfort and may require complicated medical treatment. Fortunately, only a small number of people are bitten by snakes annually. It is particularly important that first aiders and hiking and camping enthusiasts who frequent areas inhabited by poisonous snakes be able to identify poisonous snakes and know how to care for snakebites. Many good sources are available to those who wish to become more knowledgeable about snakes, their habits and dangers.

Indicators of Pit Viper Snakebite

1. Severe burning pain and swelling.
2. Dark-purplish coloring of skin.
3. Two puncture marks are usually found, although occasionally only one is located, especially if fingers or toes are bitten.
4. Growing weakness.
5. Nausea and vomiting.
6. Shortness of breath.

Indicators of Coral Snakebite

1. Similar to indicators of pit vipers, but there is no swelling and no fang marks.
2. Great drowsiness leading to rapid unconsciousness.

First Aid Procedures for Snakebites

The first aider should see to it that the individual bitten by a poisonous snake is transported to a medical facility as soon as possible. Bites about the face, neck, and trunk are especially dangerous. Studies are being made to develop new methods of care for snakebite that can be undertaken by first aiders prior to medical attention. The standard procedure for handling snakesbites is as follows:

Figure 4.9 POISONOUS SNAKES FOUND IN THE UNITED STATES

COPPERHEAD
ALSO CALLED:
HIGHLAND MOCCASIN, RATTLESNAKE PILOT, COPPERSNAKE, AND CHUNKHEAD
FOUND: Massachusetts to northern Florida; westward to Mississippi River in Illinois and across to Texas. Found in hilly, rocky country and in lowlands; in walls, hedges, slab sawdust piles, haystakcs, barns, and even in villages and towns.
SIZE: Up to 53 inches; average 3 feet.

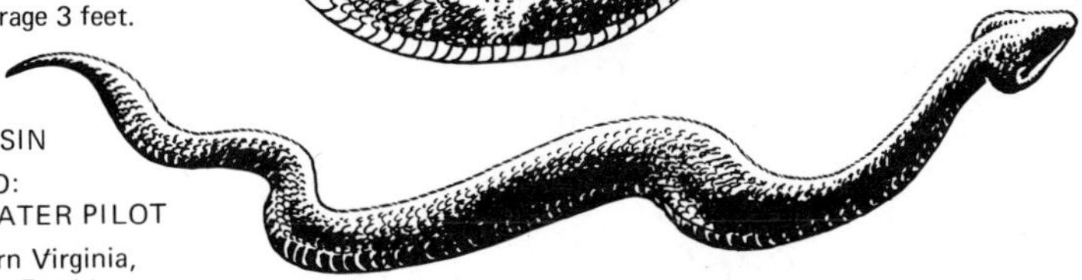

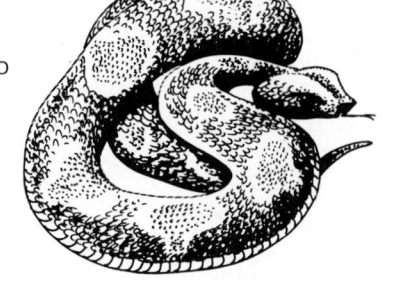

WATER MOCCASIN
ALSO CALLED:
COTTONMOUTH AND WATER PILOT
FOUND: From southeastern Virginia, along coastal plains through Florida, westward to Texas, and up the Mississippi Valley to Indiana.
SIZE: Up to 39 inches.

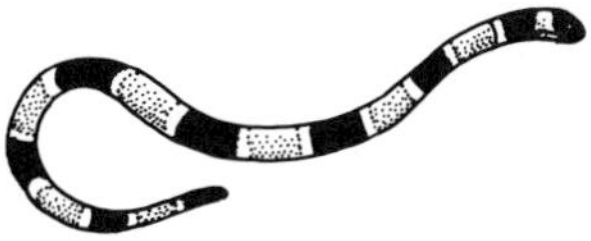

CORAL SNAKE
ALSO CALLED:
HARLEQUIN AND BEAD SNAKE
FOUND: Along the coastal plains from central North Carolina, through Florida, westward to Texas, and up the Mississippi Valley to Indiana.
SIZE: Up to 39 inches.

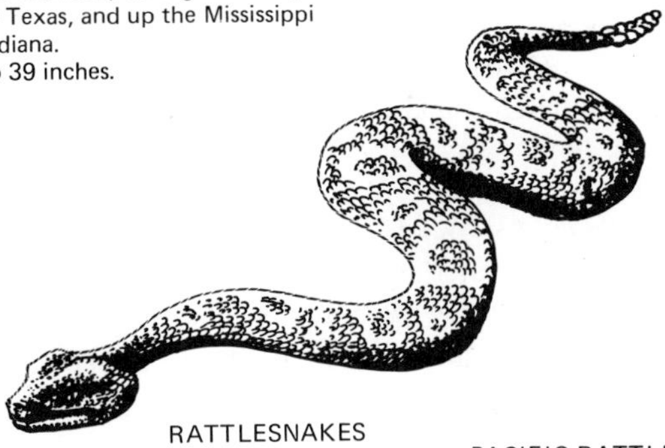

RATTLESNAKES

TIMBER
ALSO CALLED:
BANDED RATTLESNAKE, MOUNTAIN RATTLER, AND BLACK RATTLER
FOUND: In uplands and mountains from southern Maine to northern Florida and westward to central Texas.
SIZE: Up to 6 feet; average 4 feet.

DIAMONDBACK
FOUND: From central coast region of North Carolina; along lower coastal plain through Florida; westward to eastern Louisiana.
SIZE: Up to 8 feet.

PACIFIC RATTLESNAKE
FOUND: British Columbia to southern California and lower California; east to Idaho, Nevada, and Arizona.
SIZE: Up to 5 feet.

MASSASAUGA
ALSO CALLED:
PIGMY RATTLESNAKE
FOUND: Western New York and northwestern Pennsylvania; westward to northeastern Kansas on the south and southeastern Minnesota on the north. A subspecies extends into Texas, Arizona, and Colorado.
SIZE: Up to 3 feet.

[74] Soft Tissue Injuries

Figure 4.10 Constricting band for snakebite.

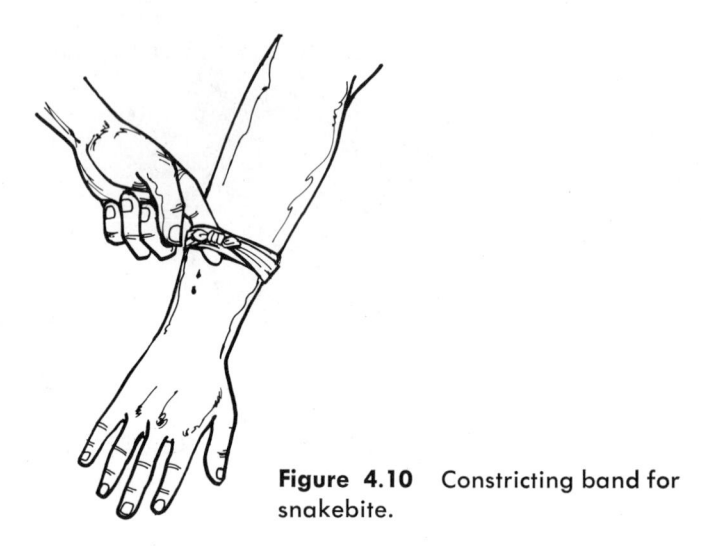

1. Stop all muscular action at once. This decreases circulatory function to some extent and thus slows the spread of the venom.
2. Apply a snug constricting band (not a tourniquet) about an inch above the bite (Figure 4.10). This should stop the flow of venous blood but not the arterial flow.
3. With a knife, razorblade, or other sharp edge, make small slashes (about ⅛ to ¼ inch deep and 2 inches long) through the fang marks in a diagonal manner or longitudinally. Be careful not to cut too deep, to avoid injuring muscles, tendons, or blood vessels.
4. Apply suction either with the mouth or the suction cup of a snakebite kit. (A first aider should not use his mouth if he has any open sore on the mouth or lips.) Suction must be done as soon as possible to be effective. It is of little use after half an hour to an hour has elapsed.
5. Keep the bite site lower than the rest of the body.
6. If swelling should spread beyond the constricting band, place another one just above it and remove the first.
7. Do not give stimulants or alcohol by mouth.
8. Transport to a medical facility as quickly as possible.

The newer method of caring for snakesbites is by cryotherapy, which consists of rapidly cooling the affected area as soon as possible after the bite. This method controls the local enzymatic destruction of the tissues involved by decreasing the activeness of the venom. In addition it slows circulation to the affected area and in turn slows the circulation of the poison to the rest of the body. This new method has proven effective for bites in the arms and legs. For snakebites in the face, neck, or trunk the standard method should be used, so as not to delay the removal of the venom.

The new cyrotherapy method of caring for snakebites is as follows:

1. Stop all muscular activity.
2. Apply a constricting band one inch above the bite site. The band is left in place until adequate cooling has been established, preferably until after the victim reaches medical attention.
3. Apply cold water or ice to the bite site. If the area can be immersed in cold water this is preferable. Observe carefully for signs of freezing. In no instance should the cold be left in contact with the bite site for longer than one hour.
4. Keep the victim warm as in caring for shock.
5. Transport to a medical facility immediately for administration of antivenom and continued cold therapy.

Human Bites

One of the most serious wounds that humans can receive are bites inflicted by other humans. Although some may be minor puncture wounds, in other cases severe lacerations may occur. The greatest danger, however, lies not in the bleeding, but in the contamination. Human bites should be cleansed thoroughly with soap and water, covered with sterile dressings, and observed carefully for signs of infection. A very severe bite or multibites may require sutures and tetanus prophylaxis; in such cases medical attention should be sought.

Animal Bites

Bites from animals (dogs, cats, rabbits, squirrels, and so on) may vary from seemingly minor puncture marks with little bleeding to severely lacerated hemorrhaging wounds. As with human bites, the danger usually lies in contamination rather than in the hemorrhage.

First Aid Procedures

1. Identify the animal that has inflicted the bite. (It is not necessary for the first aider to attempt capture of the animal; only get a description from the bitten individual, while his memory is still sharp.)
2. Control hemorrhage in severely bleeding bites.
3. Cleanse the bite area thoroughly with soap and water. Preferably soak the area and continue this en route to a medical facility. If this is not possible, cover the area with thick sterile dressings and immobilize.

4. Seek medical attention as quickly as possible.
5. Report the bite to the police or local health authorities.

The grave danger in an animal bite is the possibility of rabies. All warm-blooded animals may transmit the disease, the virus being transmitted via the saliva of the animal. The animal must be identified or captured so that it may be checked for previous rabies vaccination or observed for a period of fifteen days for signs of rabies. If the animal appears berserk and destruction is necessary, the brain may be examined for signs of the virus by the local or state health department. If it is suspected that an individual has been bitten by a rabid animal and especially if the animal cannot be located for observation, as is the case with small wild animals (rabbits, foxes, squirrels, and so on), the victim must undergo a series of injections known as the Pasteur treatment or hyperimmune serum. Treatment must be begun before the symptoms of the disease appear, or it will be ineffective. Several factors influence the necessity for these injections and the type which is to be used. As this can only be determined by the physician, it is imperative that the individual bitten by an animal seek immediate medical attention.

5

SHOCK

The word *shock* is used in association with several unrelated conditions. We speak, for example, of electrical shock, insulin shock, and anaphylactic shock, although these types are not related forms of shock. When used by itself, however, the term *shock* usually refers to a depressed body condition known medically as *traumatic shock*. Traumatic shock is a condition which demands attention apart from and regardless of the severity of the injuries incurred. Even minor injuries can trigger the autonomic nervous system in some individuals and cause them to go into shock. Shock occurs in various manners within the body, depending on the initiating source. The most common types of shock observed by first aiders are traumatic, cardiogenic, anaphylactic, emotional, psychogenic, neurogenic, and electrical. Individuals who are (1) suffering from illness, (2) fatigued, (3) emotionally upset, or (4) elderly are particularly susceptible to shock and should be given special consideration by the first aider.

TRAUMATIC SHOCK

Traumatic shock is a slowing down of the vital body processes. It is caused by a deficiency of total blood circulation due to external loss through hemorrhage, loss of plasma through wounds or burns, or dehydration caused by (1) extreme perspiration, (2) lack of water intake, (3) excess urination, (4) vomiting, (5) diarrhea, or (6) any combination of the foregoing. A normal person can lose 10 percent of his blood volume with no

[78]   Shock

apparent harm. A blood loss of 15 to 20 percent (up to two pints) will cause moderate shock, while a loss of 40 percent or over (4 pints or more) will cause severe shock and possibly death.

Traumatic shock may also be caused by internal hemorrhage as a result of crushing injuries. In this case blood collects in the body cavities and becomes unavailable for circulation.

Venous pooling—the stagnation of blood in the large veins of the body—may also cause a decrease in circulating blood volume. Blood vessels both inside and outside the body organs, especially in the abdominal cavity, may lose their vasomotor tone (a loss of normal tension resulting

Figure 5.1   CYCLIC EFFECTS OF TRAUMATIC SHOCK

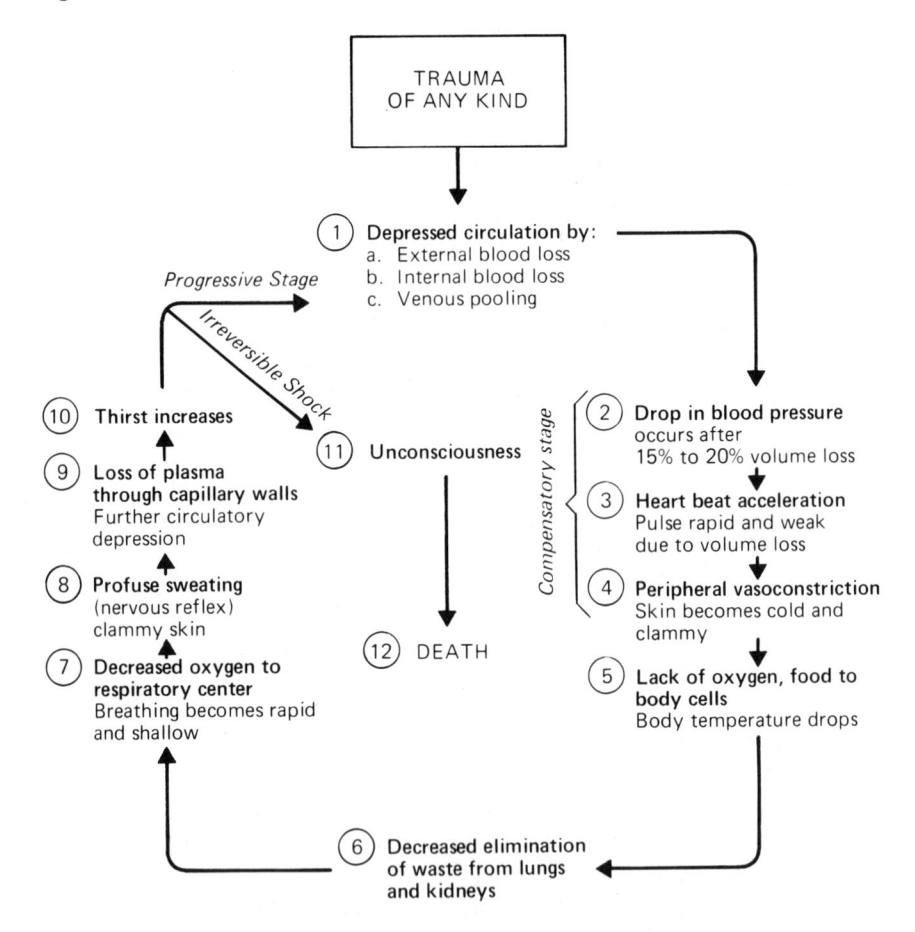

TRAUMA OF ANY KIND

1. Depressed circulation by:
   a. External blood loss
   b. Internal blood loss
   c. Venous pooling

Progressive Stage

Irreversible Shock

2. Drop in blood pressure occurs after 15% to 20% volume loss

3. Heart beat acceleration Pulse rapid and weak due to volume loss

4. Peripheral vasoconstriction Skin becomes cold and clammy

5. Lack of oxygen, food to body cells Body temperature drops

6. Decreased elimination of waste from lungs and kidneys

7. Decreased oxygen to respiratory center Breathing becomes rapid and shallow

8. Profuse sweating (nervous reflex) clammy skin

9. Loss of plasma through capillary walls Further circulatory depression

10. Thirst increases

11. Unconsciousness

12. DEATH

Compensatory stage (2–5)

Source: William T. Brennan and Donald J. Ludwig, *Guide to Problems and Practices in First Aid and Civil Defense*, 2nd ed. William C. Brown Company, Dubuque, Iowa, 1970.

Shock [79]

in a relaxation of the vessel walls) and thus increase in diameter allowing blood to collect or pool. The blood pressure drops and the gradient necessary to return blood to the heart is greatly diminished. Venous pooling may also be caused by impulses from the autonomic nervous system, or from cessation of such impulses as in fainting and emotional shock, or spinal cord and brain injuries.

As a result of this decreased blood volume, the peripheral vessels of the skin and extremities constrict (vasoconstriction) in order to provide more blood for the vital organs. In addition there is an increase in blood concentration causing a decrease in blood pressure. With the fall in blood pressure comes a further decrease in circulation, resulting in deficient oxygenation (anoxia) of the vital organs. At this point the individual's life is threatened and he is said to be in irreversible shock (Figure 5.1). Shock immediately precedes death and is one of the stages of the dying process. It is most important, then, that individuals suspected of being in shock be recognized and cared for immediately.

Indicators of Traumatic Shock

If the following indicators are present, the individual is definitely in shock and care should begin immediately.

1. Pulse is very rapid (over 100 beats per minute) but quite weak, often impossible to feel.
2. Facial skin is pale or cyanotic (bluish). In dark-skinned individuals (especially blacks) look for blueness of the lips and tongue, mucous membranes, and fingernail beds.
3. Extremities are pale and cool; skin is moist.
4. Eyes are vacant, lackluster, pupils dilated.
5. Blood pressure drops (determined by use of blood pressure cuff and stethoscope).

Any of the following signs may also be present in shock:

1. Shallow, irregular respiration.
2. Thirst.
3. Nausea and vomiting.
4. Perspiration.
5. Restlessness.
6. Large visible amounts of blood or fluid loss.

First Aid Procedures for Shock

In serious injuries, caring for shock should take priority over other first aid measures, with the exceptions of massive hemorrhage, stoppage of breathing, or cardiac arrest. In the procedures for shock outlined below, it is assumed that hemorrhage has been controlled and that an open airway has been established and maintained (see Chapters 2 and 3). There are four important points to remember in the handling of shock: (1) position, (2) temperature, (3) fluids, and (4) pain.

1. *Position—Keep the injured individual lying down.*

The best position to place an individual in shock is lying down on his back with the legs elevated 12 to 16 inches. This helps the flow of venous blood returning to the heart. The legs can be elevated by placing pillows or other objects under them (Figure 5.2).

If the injured individual is suffering from head injuries, open chest wounds, breathing difficulties, cardiac problems, or fractures to the lower extremities, elevate the head and chest. If he has neck or back injuries or complains of pain when any elevation is attempted, keep him in a flat position. Often it may be best to leave the individual in the position found, especially in collision and fall injuries where the probability of spinal injury is high.

2. *Temperature—Conserve body heat.*

The overall objective here is to conserve the injured individual's body heat by covering him with a blanket or blankets. If he is lying on the cold ground, carefully place a blanket beneath him, if this is feasible.

Care should be taken not to overheat the individual. Use of hot water bottles, heating pads, and the like should be avoided. If the surrounding temperature is very low, other sources of heat may be used, provided that extreme care is taken not to burn the individual. Excessive heat may cause the blood vessels of the skin to dilate and lose more blood from circulation. Generally speaking, then, conserve existing body heat—do not add heat unless the surrounding temperature is very low.

3. *Fluids—Restore lost body fluids.*

Although it is essential in the initial care and later definitive treatment of shock that fluid balance be rapidly restored, the first aider is not in a position to attempt this, because the only way he can give fluids is by mouth. Fluids should never be given by mouth to an injured individual who is semi-conscious, unconscious, or just regaining consciousness. Furthermore, if fluid is present in the stomach it may be necessary to postpone anesthesia and corrective surgery. It is best that the first aider not concern himself with fluid restoration. However, if the injured individual is fully conscious and medical care will be delayed two or more hours, fluids may be given. These fluids should be plain water at room temperature, or a salt and water solution (one teaspoon salt per quart of water), and should be taken by the injured slowly in sips. Never offer

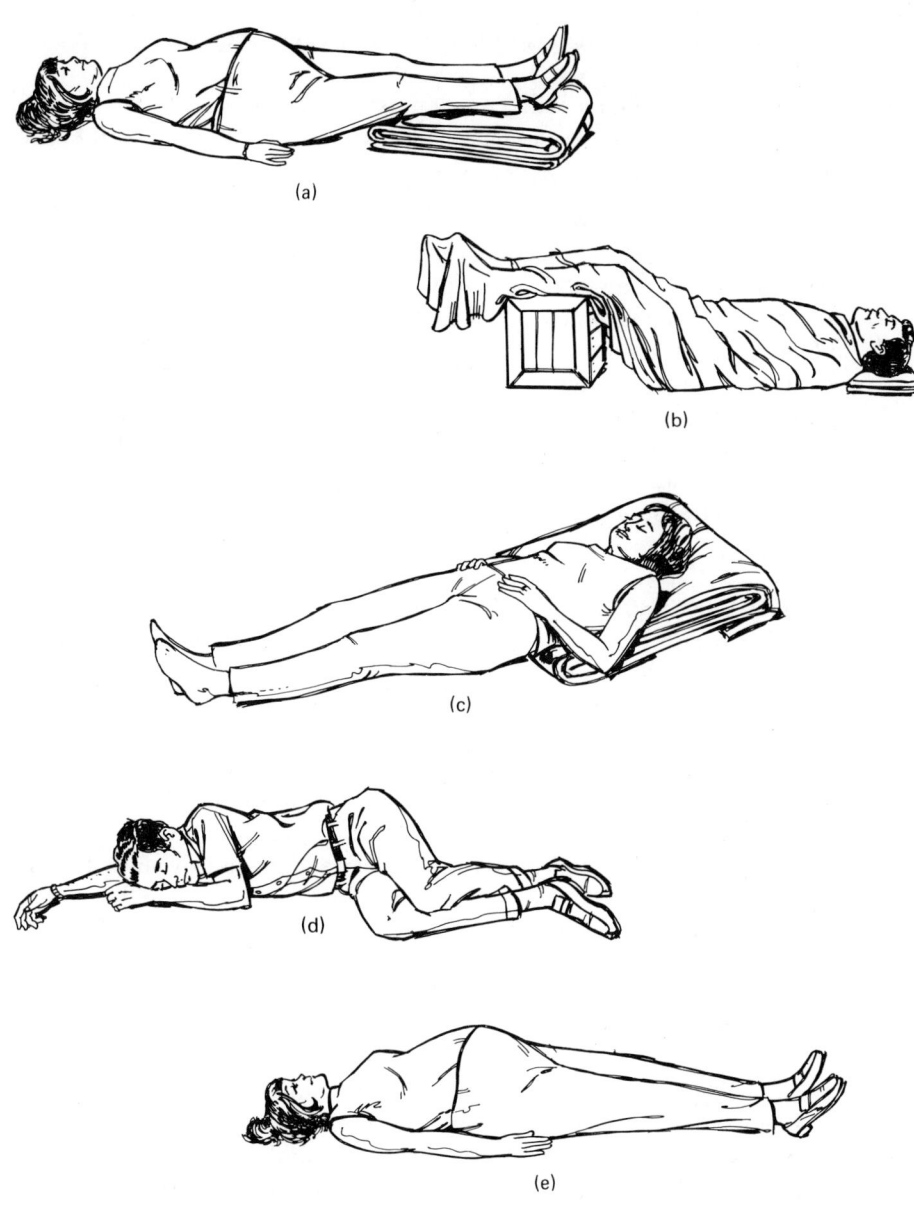

Figure 5.2 Positions for traumatic shock. To improve the circulation, individuals suspected of being in shock are usually positioned with feet elevated, as in (a) and (b). If the individual is having respiratory difficulty the head and shoulders should be elevated (c). If the individual is unconscious, he should be placed on his side (d). And if circumstances dictate, the individual should be left in the position found (e).

[81]

alcohol or stimulants such as coffee or tea, because they will only further upset the body physiology.

The necessary fluids will be administered intravenously by medical personnel (doctor, nurse, or ambulance attendant) as soon as they become available.

4. *Pain—Decrease pain.*

Pain may deepen shock, so any measure which can be taken to alleviate pain will also lessen the severity of shock. Pain may be lessened by properly bandaging open wounds, immobilizing suspected fractures, avoiding rough handling, and moving the injured individual as little as possible. It is not the role of the first aider to administer aspirin or other pain-relieving drugs. In case of severe injuries it is best to leave the individual where you find him (unless there is a danger of fire, oncoming traffic, etc.), and let a trained rescue squad or ambulance crew do the moving and transporting.

CARDIOGENIC SHOCK

Cardiogenic shock occurs after an individual suffers a severe heart attack. It is caused by a decreased effectiveness of the heart's pumping action which causes the blood pressure to drop. This drop causes an oxygen decrease to the tissue which then results in tissue death. An individual in cardiogenic shock shows the same signs as in traumatic shock. There is, however, little a first aider can do other than to recognize this condition. The individual needs medical attention quickly and it is the first aider's responsibility to see that an ambulance is called without delay to transport the individual to a medical facility.

ANAPHYLACTIC SHOCK

Anaphylactic shock develops when an individual comes in contact with a foreign protein substance (known as the *allergen*) to which he has become sensitized. These substances can very rapidly cause a violent allergic reaction. Anaphylactic shock should be considered a true emergency because death may result suddenly from respiratory collapse unless counteractant medications are administered. Individuals generally suffer anaphylactic reactions from one of four sources: (1) injection of drugs such as tetanus antitoxin or penicillin; (2) ingestion of foods such as shellfish or berries, or oral drugs; (3) insect stings such as bees, wasps, yellow jackets or hornets; and (4) inhaled substances such as dust or pollens. With the absorption of the allergen into the body, histamine is released and circulated. This causes vasodilation, venus pooling, and a diminished venous blood return, as previously discussed under traumatic shock.

Indicators of Anaphylaxis

Anaphylactic reactions may occur within a few seconds of exposure to the allergen, or may be delayed as long as thirty minutes or more. Some reactions are very rapid and severe, especially those associated with insect stings and inhaled substances. An individual who is suffering from apparent anaphylactic shock may exhibit the following indicators:

1. Hives over a large part of the body.
2. Restlessness.
3. Itching or burning skin, especially about the chest and face.
4. Tightening or pain in the chest; wheezing.
5. Tingling sensation in the extremities, especially the fingers and toes.
6. Congestion of fluid in the lungs.
7. Edema (swelling) of the vocal cords resulting in gasping, breathing difficulty, and eventual cyanosis.
8. Collapse, similar to deep shock.
9. Unconsciousness and eventual death.

Not all of the above indicators are always present, since individuals react differently to different substances. However, if the signs indicate anaphylactic shock, the individual should receive proper care as quickly as possible.

First Aid Procedures for Anaphylaxis

Anaphylactic shock is a real emergency. There must be no delay in getting the individual to a hospital, preferably by ambulance. While waiting for the ambulance and during transport the first aider should proceed as follows:

1. If the individual is breathing, place him in a semi-reclining position to ease breathing; give care for shock.
2. If the condition is a result of a bee or wasp sting in an extremity, place a constricting band between the sting and the heart, and scrape out the stinger with your fingernail, a needle, or a knife.
3. If respiration ceases, begin and continue mouth-to-mouth artificial ventilation.

EMOTIONAL SHOCK

Upon witnessing a horrible accident, or from extreme pain, fear, anxiety, or the receipt of shocking news, a person may experience an emotional trauma. The reaction may be immediate or may occur hours or even days later.

Since the autonomic nervous system can trigger venous pooling of blood, the individual in emotional shock may appear as about to faint or may actually lapse into shock. In this situation the first aider should care for the individual as he would for fainting or shock. On the other hand, the individual may react by becoming emotionally uncontrollable, even to the point of hysteria. This requires a different avenue of approach. More and more the first aider needs to be aware of such emotional occurrences and to be prepared to help these individuals, while at the same time realizing his own limitations. Individuals injured emotionally need medical attention just as much as those who are injured physically. A more detailed and specific discussion of emotional shock and psychological first aid is given in Chapter 10.

PSYCHOGENIC SHOCK (FAINTING)

Psychogenic shock, or fainting, is one of the most common first aid emergencies. It generally occurs suddenly, with a partial or complete loss of consciousness. Fainting results from anoxia (lack of oxygen) in the brain, which is often caused by venous pooling (stagnation of blood in the large veins). It may be brought on by fright, sudden news (either good or bad), the sight of blood, injury, or death. A person can faint from severe pain or from the dread of anticipated pain, as before medical treatment. Prolonged standing in one spot may result in fainting, as may getting up abruptly from a prone or seated position.

Particularly susceptible to fainting are individuals who have been confined in a hot, stuffy atmosphere; individuals who are not feeling well; and individuals who are tired, worried, or have not eaten for some time.

Indicators of Psychogenic Shock

Prior to complete collapse, individuals almost always exhibit a similar set of signs and symptoms. They may become nauseous, begin yawning, or feel lightheaded. The face becomes quite pale and, along with the limbs, is generally covered with perspiration. They feel a tingling or numbness in the extremities, things turn black, and they slump into unconsciousness.

Shock

First Aid Procedures

Unless caused by serious medical complications such as a heart attack or stroke, fainting is a self-correcting condition. Once sufficient oxygen reaches the brain, consciousness returns. If the individual does not regain consciousness within a short period of time or if he continues to relapse into unconsciousness, seek medical attention immediately. A more serious condition may be causing the unconsciousness, not simple fainting.

In cases of simple fainting proceed as follows:

1. If the individual has already passed out, place him on his back with the feet elevated 12 to 16 inches (Figure 5.3a). This will facilitate the venous return to the heart. Keep him in this position for at least ten minutes. If he gets up too quickly he may again lose consciousness.
2. If the individual is feeling faint but is still on his feet, he should be seated and his head lowered between his knees (Figure 5.3b). This will replenish the oxygen supply to the brain and prevent complete loss of consciousness.
3. Cool wet cloths applied to the forehead and face may be comforting, but do not flood the face with water. Fresh air is vital, so the first aider should see that onlookers are kept at a distance.
4. Ammonia inhalants and stimulants should not be used indiscriminately as they may do more harm than good. Never use them on an individual who has suffered an apparent heart attack or stroke. Normally an individual will regain consciousness upon being placed in a reclining position with feet raised, without the need for spirits of ammonia. If, however, he does not, transport to a medical facility immediately.

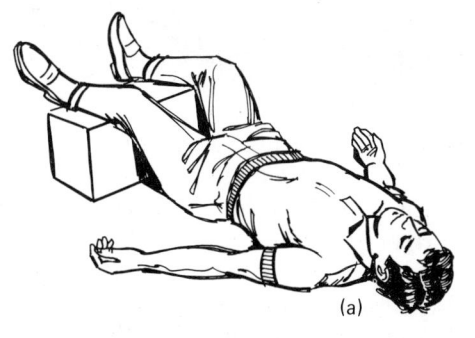

Figure 5.3 If an individual has fainted, lay him down with his feet elevated 12 to 16 inches (a). If the individual is feeling faint or is about to pass out, seat him on a chair and place his head between his knees (b).

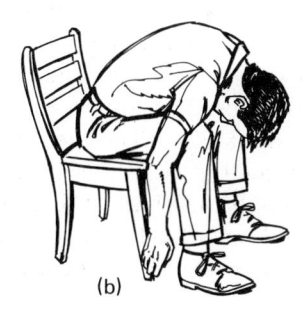

NEUROGENIC SHOCK

Venous pooling can also occur to individuals who have suffered damage to the central nervous system, as in brain and spinal injuries. Impulse pathways to the veins are interrupted, causing loss of vasomotor tone and pooling. These individuals appear as though they are in traumatic shock and should be cared for in the same manner. It is imperative that they not be moved indiscriminately due to the injury to the central nervous system.

SHOCK CAUSED BY ELECTRICAL CONTACT

With the ever-increasing use of electrical devices has come a potential source of death. Handled properly, electricity is quite safe; handled indiscriminately, it can cause sudden cardiopulmonary arrest and ultimate death. In most instances electrical shocks are a direct result of carelessness or neglect.

Several factors can affect the severity of electrical shock: the voltage and amperage, the type of contact with the electrical current, and the location where the current enters the body. Moisture from perspiration, rain, or standing water will increase the severity of the shock, as will contact with certain metals. Insulating and nonconducting materials such as dry wood or rubber will drastically reduce conductance and the possibility of shock. If the current enters through one leg while the other leg remains on the ground, the current will usually seek ground through the easiest pathway—in this case the other leg—thus probably not causing severe internal damage since it has avoided passing through the entire body, especially the heart and brain. This would not hold true, however, when current enters through the hands and leaves through the leg, as it often does in accidental electrocutions.

The damage to the body caused by electricity varies considerably. Third degree burns will appear at the point of entrance and exit of the current. However, these external burns should not be of immediate concern to the first aider. Because current generally follows blood vessel pathways it may also cause extensive burning of these tissues. Nerves located close to these vessels are also burned by the current. The greatest internal damage associated with electrical shock results when the current paralyzes the respiratory and circulatory centers of the brain, causing cardiopulmonary arrest or ventricular fibrillation (a twitching of the individual heart muscle fibers, causing ineffective pumping of the heart). Both conditions require immediate emergency first aid.

Indicators of Electrical Shock

The circumstances of the accident are the most obvious indication of an electrical shock. The injured may have been struck by lightning during an electrical storm or have come in contact with an electrical current via an appliance, plug, or exposed wire. (Physicians claim that an individual struck by lightning can withstand anoxia longer and is more easily resuscitated than one suffering from other types of electrical shock.) When the first aider arrives, the injured individual may or may not still be in contact with the current. Additional indications of electrical shock are: (1) absence of breathing, (2) weak or absent pulse, (3) dilated pupils, and (4) cyanosis. Also present, as mentioned above, are the burns at the point of entrance and exit of the current.

First Aid Procedures for Electrical Shock

Electrical shock is a real emergency and should be dealt with as such. The first aider himself should be careful to avoid suffering an electrical shock when he tries to help the injured individual.

1. Before touching the injured individual, remove him from the source of electrical current. This may be accomplished by simply turning off the current at the switch. If this is impossible, stand on a dry board or dry, nonconducting material such as rubber, and pull the individual away from the contact, using one hand that has been protected with nonconducting insulated materials (Figure 5.4). Extreme care on the part of the

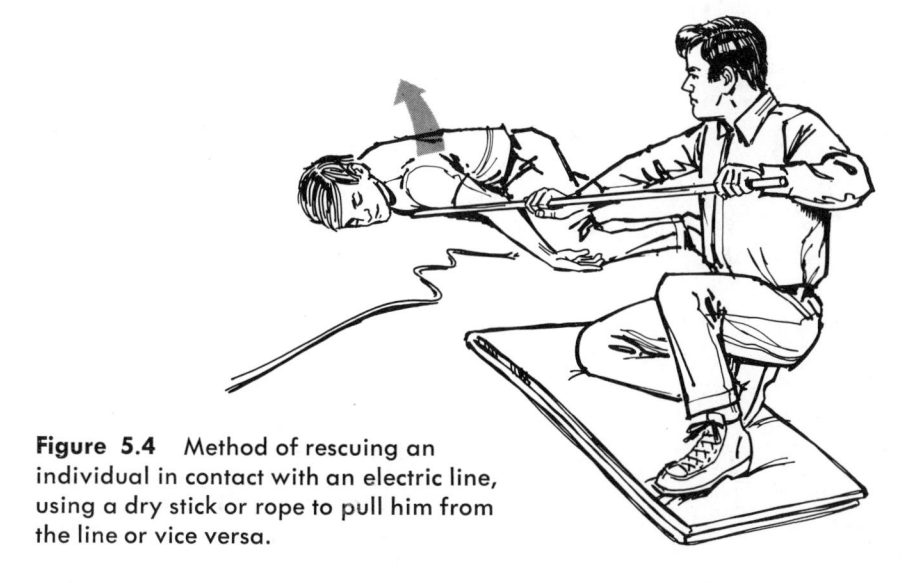

Figure 5.4 Method of rescuing an individual in contact with an electric line, using a dry stick or rope to pull him from the line or vice versa.

first aider in carrying out this rescue is imperative for self-protective purposes.
2. Once the victim is removed from contact, begin cardiopulmonary resuscitation immediately. Continue resuscitation until the individual begins to breathe or is pronounced dead by medical personnel.
3. Once resuscitated, and while being transported to a hospital, observe the injured individual, as traumatic shock often develops. Also, electrical shock victims, upon successful resuscitation, may attempt to run about or act in a disoriented manner. The first aider must, in the best way possible, protect the injured individual from harming himself. Medical attention should always be sought following severe electrical shock.

{ 6 }

SKELETAL SYSTEM INJURIES

Bone injuries are those which involve the skeletal structure of the body.* More specifically, they include fractures, sprains, strains, and dislocations. Seldom are these injuries severe enough to be considered life-threatening; however, if not cared for initially, they could result in permanent disability. Further complications—shock, injury to soft tissue, blood vessels, and nerves—are often associated with fractures. Additional damage is often inflicted upon the injured individual when well-intentioned bystanders try to help, but actually do more damage by improperly moving him. Perhaps one of the most important principles in the care of fractures can be found in the popular phrase, "Splint 'em where they lie." With proper splinting completed the injured individual can be moved comfortably, thus minimizing the danger of inflicting further injury.

CAUSES OF FRACTURES

Fractures generally occur as a result of one or more of the following circumstances: (1) a direct blow, (2) an indirect blow, (3) opposing forces, and (4) strong muscular contractions.

A direct blow to the bone will cause the bone to fracture at the site of the blow. An indirect blow will cause the bone to break some distance from the actual point of impact. An indirect blow most often occurs when

---

*For the anatomy of the skeletal system, see Appendix A.

[90] Skeletal System Injuries

a person falls, bracing himself with his hands. Due to the straight elbow, the forces of the blow travel up the arm and ultimately fracture the clavicle (collarbone).

When strong opposing forces are applied to bone ends, the forces tend to bend the bone beyond its breaking point where it gives way. Fortunately the first aider will seldom encounter fractures of this kind.

In rare instances the force of a contracting muscle can twist or tear a bone or cause a piece of bone to break off at the site. Fractures of the ankle frequently occur in this manner.

Most fractures occur as a result of automobile collisions, falls, athletic activities, and accidents in the home, all of which provide the forces or blows described above. The first aider must suspect fractures in these situations even though the obvious indicators may not appear.

TYPES OF FRACTURES

A fracture is any break in a bone, complete or incomplete, or loss of normal bone continuity. The two broad classifications of fractures are closed fractures and open fractures. This category can generally be determined by simple observation.

A *closed fracture* is one where the bone has not perforated the skin and there is no surface wound associated with the fracture area (Figure 6.1).

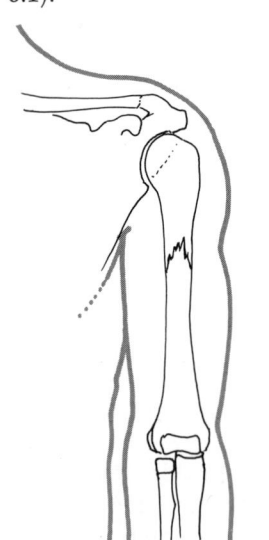

Figure 6.1 Closed fracture.

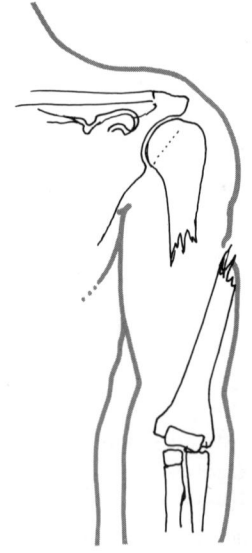

Figure 6.2 Open fracture.

An *open fracture* (formerly called a *compound fracture*) is one where a wound is associated with the fracture area (Figure 6.2). The wound may have been caused by the bone end piercing the skin or by a foreign object, such as a bullet, entering from the outside. The bone end may be protruding through the open wound or it may have receded. Regardless of the circumstances of the injury, an open wound will be evident and hemorrhage may occur if blood vessels have been damaged.

Through the use of X-rays, fractures can be classified more specifically into the following types (Figure 6.3):

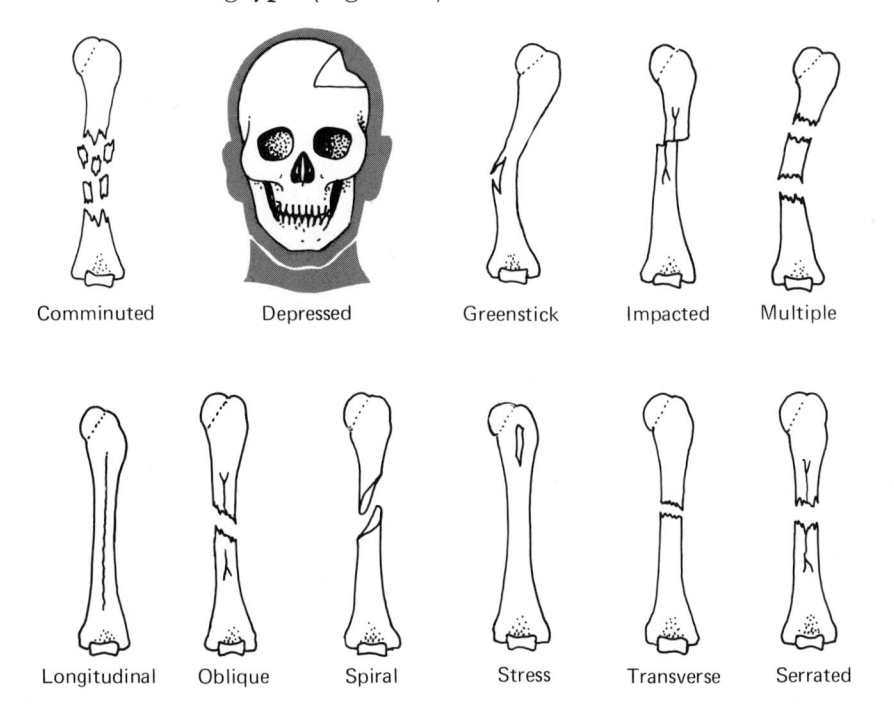

Comminuted Depressed Greenstick Impacted Multiple

Longitudinal Oblique Spiral Stress Transverse Serrated

Figure 6.3 Common types of fractures.

1. *Comminuted.* A comminuted fracture usually results from a direct blow to the bone, causing it to break into three or more bone fragments.
2. *Depressed.* A depressed fracture occurs as a result of a blow to the flat bones of the body such as those of the skull and pelvis. The danger with this type of fracture is not in the break itself, but in the resultant injury to soft body tissue.
3. *Greenstick.* When the bone is not completely calcified, as in children, the break is incomplete, or what is termed a greenstick fracture.
4. *Impacted.* Impacted fractures often occur to the long bones as a result of falling from a height. Due to the force of the fall, the bone ends

overlap or jam into each other. Medically applied traction may be required for proper healing to occur.
5. *Multiple.* The term multiple fractures is used when a bone is broken in several places or when there are fractures in several bones (for example, the humerus, the femur, and the clavicle).
6. *Longitudinal.* In a longitudinal fracture the break occurs along the long axis of the bone, with little separation occurring.
7. *Oblique.* The break in an oblique fracture occurs diagonally across the bone. Movement of this type of fracture could result in nerve or blood vessel damage due to the jagged bone ends. With mishandling it may easily become an open fracture.
8. *Spiral.* Spiral fractures are similar to longitudinal fractures in that they occur along the long axis of the bone. However, they appear as an S-shaped break, usually occurring when the foot is firmly planted and a rotating force is applied in an opposing direction, as in skiing.
9. *Stress.* Stress fractures occur as a result of a weakened or diseased bone or due to a sudden, violent muscular contraction.
10. *Transverse.* Unlike oblique fractures, transverse fractures break at right angles to the long axis of the bone. As in the oblique fracture, there is danger of nerve and blood vessel damage.
11. *Serrated.* In a serrated fracture the bone ends are jagged and uneven. Movement of the bone ends may result in nerve and blood vessel damage.

INDICATORS OF FRACTURES

There are several signs and symptoms to indicate the existence of a fracture, but all need not always be present. Often a first aider will not suspect a fracture when one actually exists, while at other times a suspected fracture may turn out to be a sprain. The first aider should always suspect and care for fractures if the injured individual—especially if elderly—receives a severe blow, falls from any height, or is thrown from a vehicle. Confirmation of fracture can usually be made through an X-ray. The first aider should be guided by the following indicators:
1. Circumstances or history of the accident.
2. The injured individual reports hearing something "pop" or "crack."
3. Pain at or near the site of the suspected fracture.
4. Tenderness on palpation of the affected area.
5. Swelling in the affected area.
6. Deformity of the affected limb, such as an unnatural position or irregularity in the continuity of the limb.
7. Pain on attempted movement.

8. Partial or complete loss of use of the extremity.
9. A grating sound or sensation (crepitus) at the site of the suspected injury.
10. Shortening of the limb. Contracting muscles may cause the bone ends to overlap, thus shortening the affected limb.
11. Bone ends visible through the open wound.

If the injured individual is conscious, it is relatively easy to ascertain a possible fracture using the indicators listed above. However, if the injured individual is unconscious, and there is reason to suspect the presence of fractures, a systematic examination of the bones may be necessary. This examination may be made quickly and easily as illustrated in Figure 6.4.

Beginning with the skull, feel with both hands all portions of the skull, checking for depressions, hemorrhage, and/or swelling. Continue on to the clavicles, moving the fingers along the bone, feeling for any separations or depressions. Continue down the arms (one at a time or simultaneously) and to the fingers. Check the sternum and ribs for depressions or abnormalities. The pelvis must be examined at the pubis as well as at the hip. Fractures in the pubic area are usually extremely painful and even slight pressure will induce signs of pain on the injured's face. Continue by examining the legs in the same manner as the arms. The vertebrae may be checked as described below under neck and back injuries.

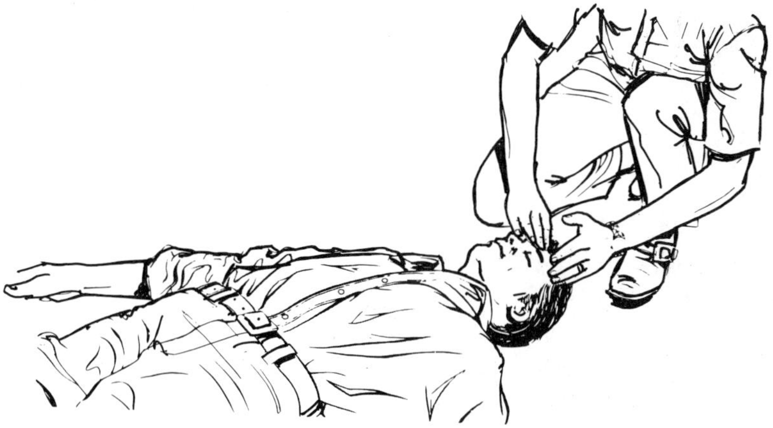

(a)

Figure 6.4 When examining a person for possible fractures, the first aider should make a systematic examination of the bony structure, feeling for depressions, protrusions, swelling, and pieces. Begin at

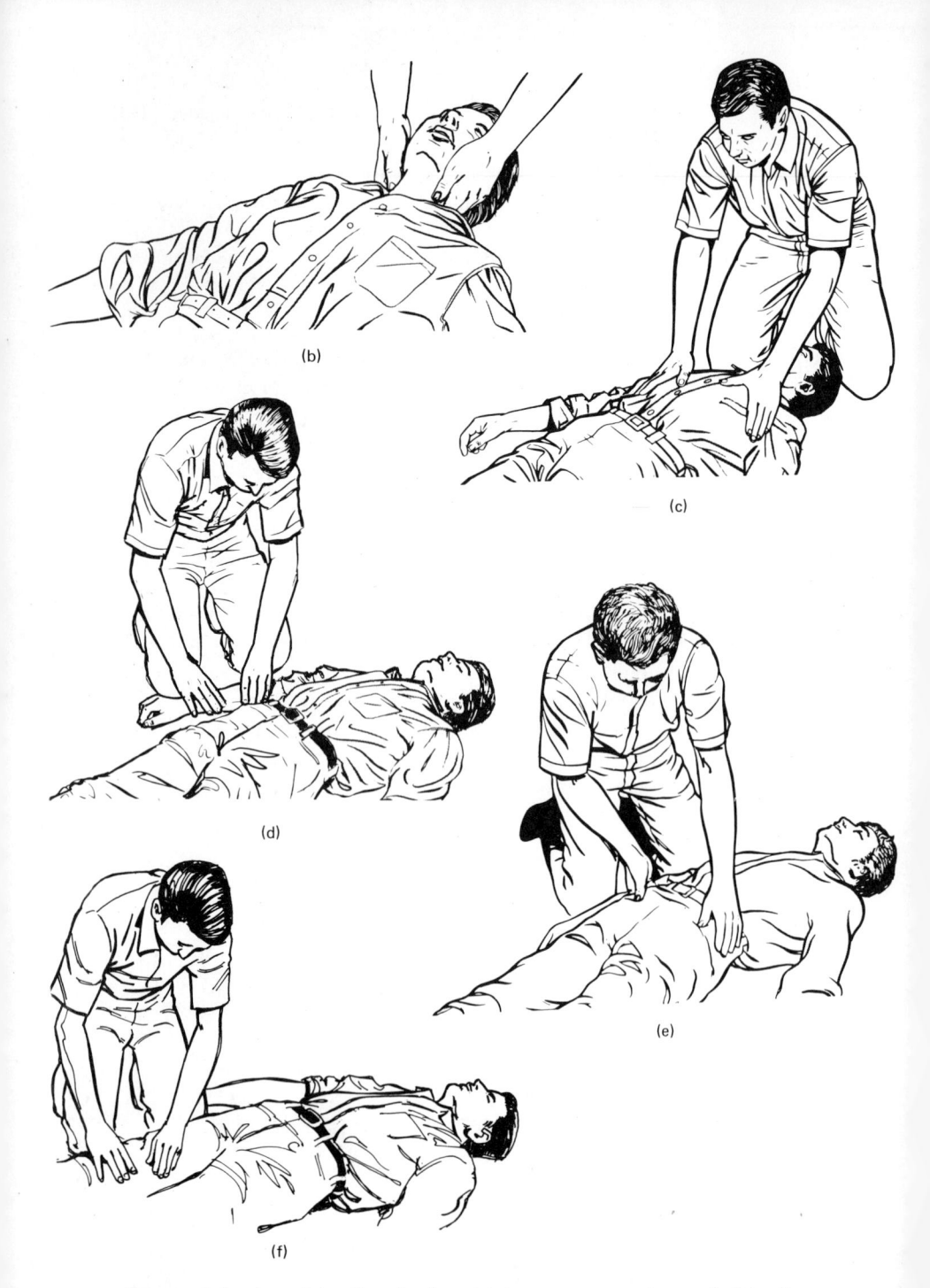

Figure 6.4 (continued) the head (a), progress to the neck (b), ribs (c), upper extremities, simultaneously or one at a time (d), pelvis (e), and finally the lower extremities, one leg at a time or simultaneously (f). This procedure should be followed whether the individual is conscious or unconscious.

PROCEDURES FOR CLOSED FRACTURES

When caring for a suspected fracture, the first aider must keep three objectives in mind: (1) prevention of bone displacement, (2) prevention of shock, and (3) relieving of pain. The injured individual should not be moved until all suspected fractures have been immobilized through the use of a fixation splint. (Exception: If the injured individual is in immediate danger due to impending fire or explosion, he must be moved, but with utmost care.) In suspected femur fractures, a traction splint may be necessary; however, traction is a paramedical procedure to be applied by an ambulance crew or at the hospital.

A variety of commercial and improvised devices may be used to splint the suspected fracture. Commercially prepared splints come in several types—cardboard, aluminum, wood, air, etc. But if these commercial devices are not available, a variety of common household items can serve to immobilize the area just as well. Folded newspapers and magazines, pillows and blankets, umbrellas, tongue depressors, cardboard, poles, baseball bats, tree limbs, and flat boards may be used. If none of these is available, simply immobilize the fracture area by securing the injured limb to the noninjured limb or portion of the body. A detailed explanation of splinting with various types of splints is given in Chapter 12. Certain general principles apply to all types.

When applying a fixation splint to a suspected fracture the first aider should be mindful of the following:

1. The splint must be long enough to immobilize the joint above and below the suspected fracture. For example, if the lower leg is fractured, the knee and ankle joints must be kept immobile.
2. Pad the splint. This is for the purposes of comfort and to provide additional protection for the injured area. Padding should be used to fill the body voids, that is, under the wrist, ankle, and behind the knee.
3. Splint the affected area in the most comfortable position for the individual. Do not attempt to straighten the affected area or to reduce the fracture in any way.
4. When securing the splint, the ties should be fastened away from the fracture site. If tied against the affected area, pressure from the knot may cause additional pain, tissue damage, or impairment of circulation.
5. The ties should be snug but not so tight as to inhibit circulation. Check periodically as the affected area may begin to swell, thus compromising circulation.
6. Do not move the injured individual until all suspected fractures are immobilized and sufficient help is available to move the individual properly.
7. Check and care for shock, keeping the injured individual in a reclining or sem-reclining position.
8. Transport to a medical facility.

PROCEDURES FOR OPEN FRACTURES

The first aid procedures for open fractures differ from closed fracture procedures in that hemorrhage at the fracture site must be controlled. Care should be taken when applying direct pressure to the wound, because it is possible to damage nerves and blood vessels which are in close proximity to the affected area. Indirect pressure may be more advantageous, depending upon the extent of the hemorrhage. Once the hemorrhage is controlled, cover the wound with a sterile dressing, splint the affected area, check and care for shock, if present, and transport to a medical facility.

SPECIAL FRACTURES

Fractures of the pelvis, skull, jaw, neck, and back require special consideration as these fractures often cause severe damage to underlying soft tissue. Skull and back fractures are especially dangerous because of the potential damage to the brain and to the delicate tissues of the spinal cord.

Pelvic Fractures

Fractures of the pelvis have become more frequent with increases in the number of automobile collisions. This type of fracture is also common among the elderly when they suffer a serious fall. When the pelvis is fractured serious complications such as injuries to the bladder, urinary tract, intestines, or reproductive organs may be present.

Indicators of Pelvic Fractures

If one or more of the following indicators are present, handle as a pelvic fracture:

1. Pain in the pelvic region following a fall or blow.
2. Signs of a strain or contusion in the pelvic area.
3. Inability of the injured individual to lift leg while lying on back.
4. Outward turning of the injured foot and leg.
5. Possible shortening of one leg.

First Aid Procedures for Pelvic Fractures

1. Immobilize the entire pelvic area with a well-padded board that reaches from the shoulders to the feet.
2. Make the injured individual as comfortable as possible.
3. Check and care for shock.
4. Transport to a medical facility.

Skull Fractures

Fractures to the skull differ from fractures of the weight-bearing bones in that the skull serves as a container for the brain and with injury serious brain damage could result. The most severe injuries occur from hemorrhage and lacerations to the brain tissue. Skull fractures can also result in the leakage of cerebrospinal fluid, or blood in severe injuries, from the ears, nose, or mouth. An injury of this type opens a channel for infection to the brain area. A depressed fracture may cause severe brain damage, especially if the fracture occurs on the back of the head causing injury to the respiratory and circulatory center of the brain.

Indicators of Skull Fractures

The first aider should suspect a skull fracture and handle accordingly if any of the following indicators exist.

1. The injured individual has received a blow to the head as a result of a fall, automobile collision, or being struck by an object, for example, a baseball bat.
2. The injured individual may be unconscious or may be regaining consciousness.
3. Watery cerebrospinal fluid or blood may be coming from the ears, nose, or mouth.
4. Pupils of the eye may be unequally dilated.

First Aid Procedures for Skull Fractures

1. Do not attempt to raise the head or place a pillow under the head. Make sure that the airway is clear, and kept open.
2. Make the injured individual as comfortable as possible in a reclining position, preferably lying on the uninjured side. This will help to relieve pressure on the injured side and allow for drainage of cerebrospinal fluids.
3. Keep the injured individual absolutely quiet and try to keep all onlookers away.
4. Do not administer any fluids by mouth.
5. Do not attempt to arouse the injured individual with the use of ammonia inhalants.
6. Check and care for shock.
7. Transport to a medical facility, preferably by ambulance.

Concussion

The brain, which is encased within the skull, may be injured without actual fracturing of the skull bones. This may occur as a result of an automobile collision or a blow by a blunt object. If the brain receives a

[98] Skeletal System Injuries

violent shaking it may be bruised, and cerebrospinal fluid may escape or actual hemorrhaging may take place. As there is only a very small space between the brain and the skull bones, the fluid pressure may accumulate on the brain, compressing blood vessels and limiting the oxygen supply to that portion of the brain. The severity of the concussion depends on the amount of fluid present and the location of the pressure of the fluid.

Indicators of a Concussion

An individual who has suffered a concussion and/or possible brain injury may exhibit a variety of indicators, among which are the following:

1. History of a fall, blow to the head, or automobile collision.
2. Possible depressed bone fracture to the skull.
3. The injured individual may or may not be conscious. If conscious, determine whether he has previously been unconscious for any period of time.
4. If conscious, the injured individual may feel faint, lightheaded or dizzy, or complain of a severe headache.
5. The pupils of the eye may be unequally dilated, possibly indicating a brain injury.
6. The injured individual may appear restless, confused, or disoriented.
7. The injured individual may be vomiting or complaining of nausea.
8. The injured individual generally exhibits the classical signs of shock.

First Aid Procedures for Concussion

The first aider should make the injured individual as comfortable as possible while caring for shock. Do not admiinster any fluids or medications. If unconscious, place the injured individual on his side with the head slightly lower than the rest of the body. Oxygen may be administered if available, and cold compresses may be applied to the head. Immediate medical attention should be sought.

Lower Jaw Fractures

Fractures to the lower jaw generally occur from a direct blow to the face, and usually a wound will be present inside of the mouth.

Indicators of a Jaw Fracture

The first aider must suspect a jaw fracture and handle for such if any of the following indicators are present:

1. Circumstance or history of the accident, for example, a blow to the face.
2. Pain on attempted movement of the jaw—difficulty in speaking.

3. Blood and/or saliva drooling from the mouth.
4. Broken or missing teeth.

First Aid Procedures for Jaw Fracture

1. Gently close the jaw so that the lower jaw rests against the upper jaw.
2. Secure with bandage. Tie with a bow knot for easy removal as the injured individual may vomit.
3. Check and care for shock.
4. Transport to a medical facility.

Spinal Fractures

A fractured vertebra is perhaps the most serious type of fracture, and correct handling of the injured individual is extremely important. The spinal cord is contained within a canal formed by the vertebrae. The vertebrae serve to protect the spinal cord from injury; however, the exertion of a great compressive force (as in an automobile or airplane crash, or a fall from a great height) will collapse and injure or compress the vertebrae causing an angulation of the spinal cord. Although the fracture itself does not present any great danger, damage can result if bone fragments injure the tissue of the spinal cord or spinal nerves. Severance or compression of the cord can result in paralysis or even ultimate death. The most common spinal fractures occur in the cervical (neck) and lumbar (lower back) vertebrae (Figure 6.5).

Because of the seriousness of spinal cord injuries, proper handling of the injured individual is extremely important. Improper movement of the injured individual can cause an increase in the curvature of the spine, resulting in further damage to the spinal cord. Individuals who have fallen or been involved in a collision should never be moved until two things have been determined: (1) Is there a possible spinal fracture? and (2) If so, where?

Indicators of Vertebral Fracture

The first aider must suspect vertebral fracture and handle accordingly if any of the following indicators are present:

1. Circumstances or history of the accident.
2. Severe pain in the neck or back area.
3. Inability to move arms or legs, or slowness in movement.
4. Weakness, numbness, or tingling sensation in the arms or legs.

If the injured individual is conscious he can help the first aider determine the location of the possible fracture by answering a few simple

[100]   Skeletal System Injuries

questions. Ask the injured individual if he can move his fingers or grasp your hand. If his grip is weak or he is unable to move his fingers, a cervical (neck) injury may be suspected. Likewise, ask him to move his feet or toes; if he is unable to do so, this suggests a lumbar (back) injury. If the injured individual is unconscious, prick the palm of the hand with a pin or sharp object; if no reflex action occurs (involuntary closing of fingers), the vertebrae of the neck may be injured. Likewise, prick the

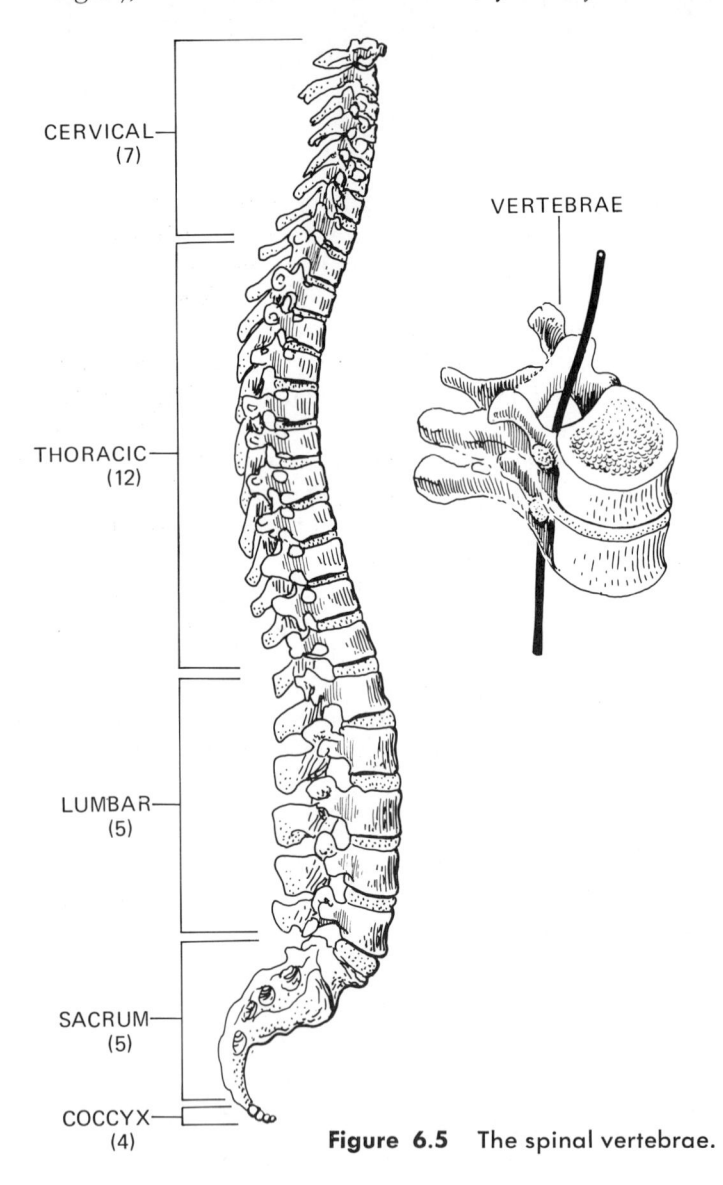

CERVICAL (7)

THORACIC (12)

VERTEBRAE

LUMBAR (5)

SACRUM (5)

COCCYX (4)

Figure 6.5 The spinal vertebrae.

Skeletal System Injuries [101]

sole of the foot or the back of the knee, and if there is no involuntary movement of the foot, injury to the lower back vertebrae is likely.

First Aid Procedures for Vertebral Fracture

Extreme care must be taken in immobilizing and transporting a suspected vertebral fracture. Immediate care for shock and immobilization on a rigid surface are required. It is advisable to wait until sufficient help arrives (via an ambulance) before moving the injured individual, otherwise serious spinal cord damage could occur. The proper techniques for immobilizing suspected vertebral fractures are discussed in detail in Chapter 12.

INJURIES RELATED TO THE SKELETAL SYSTEM

Often when an individual falls or is struck by a heavy object the bone may not be injured sufficiently to actually break. However, the stress placed on the skeletal structure may result in injuries to the joints and/or muscles of this system. These injuries are handled as suspected fractures until proven otherwise by an X-ray.

Sprains

Sprains are injuries to the soft tissues (ligaments and tendons) which surround a joint. Sprains may occur at any joint in the body, the most common being at the ankle.

Indicators of a Sprain

Sprains occur when the joint is forced beyond its normal range of movement. Most are caused by a sudden twisting or wrenching motion. The indicators are like those of a fracture and are distinguished from a fracture only through an X-ray. Pain, swelling, discoloration, tenderness, and loss of movement are usually present.

First Aid Procedures for Sprains

The object is to prevent swelling and hemorrhage in the affected joint.

1. Elevate the affected joint if possible.
2. Apply ice to the affected joint.
3. Immobilize the affected joint as a fracture.
4. Check and care for shock.
5. Transport to a medical facility.

Dislocations

Like sprains, dislocations also occur at the joints of the body. Due to a sudden stretching, twisting, or jerking, the bone ends become displaced. They may be pulled apart, overlapped, or become parallel to one another.

Indicators of a Dislocation

A dislocated joint shows the same signs as a suspected fracture and should be handled as such until proven otherwise by an x-ray. The unnatural shape of the joint is the most prominent indicator, along with pain, discoloration, and loss of movement.

First Aid Procedures for Dislocations

Proper alignment of the bone ends may require surgery, and the first aider should not attempt to reduce any dislocation. Attempted or even improper alignment may result in nerve, soft tissue or blood vessel injury, or a permanent deformity. Therefore, the first aider should handle dislocations as suspected fractures.

1. Immobilize the affected joint.
2. Apply ice to the affected joint.
3. Check and care for shock.
4. Transport to a medical facility.

Strains

Strains differ from sprains and dislocations in that they do not affect the bony structure of the body, but rather involve the muscles which allow for body movement. Strains result when a muscle or a group of muscles are overstretched. Injury to the muscle may be quite mild, as in simple overexertion, or serious enough to actually tear the muscle fibers with resultant hemorrhage. Strains usually occur as a result of a sudden, violent movement, most often when lifting a heavy object or exercising unused muscles.

Indicators of a Strain

The injured individual will complain of a sharp pain or a burning sensation in the affected muscle, or of feeling something snap within the muscle. Severe weakness or even loss of function may occur. Tenderness is complained of on palpation, and in severe strains a dislocation may also be present.

First Aid Procedures for Strains

1. At the time of the injury, apply ice and compression with an elastic bandage. Continue this for 24 hours, so as to lessen any hemorrhage which may occur.
2. After 24 hours, apply moist heat to absorb the hemorrhage.
3. Rest the affected muscles.
4. Seek medical attention if the pain is severe or persists.

{ 7 }

BURNS AND EXPOSURE

When the human body is exposed to extremes in environmental temperatures it has the capacity to adjust, but this adjustment takes a period of time. When people are not accustomed to temperature extremes and are suddenly exposed to extreme heat or cold conditions, their body does not have time to adjust and it may become injured. The most common cold-associated injury is frostbite which, if severe enough, may result in the loss of extremities such as toes or fingers. Heat has varying effects upon the body, depending on the source and length of exposure. One may receive a burn from a direct heat source, inhale superheated air, become exhausted by heat, develop muscle cramps, or, more seriously, suffer from a heat stroke—all as a result of exposure to a heated environment. Prevention plays a decisive role in counteracting ill effects of heat and cold upon the body. Precautionary measures include learning to dress properly so as to reflect or conserve body heat, to regulate exercise and length of exposure, and, of course, to prevent fires.

ADVERSE EFFECTS OF HEAT

As previously stated, heat may affect the body in various ways. Direct burns are painful regardless of how deep or how extensive. Environmental effects from exposure include heat exhaustion, heat cramps, and heat stroke, the latter being the most severe. Almost everyone who works or plays in a hot, humid environment has experienced heat exhaustion or possibly heat cramps. Football trainers and coaches have learned that periodic rests and saline liquids are needed during late spring and early fall practice to prevent severe heat complications among the players. Lifeguards and sun-worshipers must be on the lookout for heat stroke effects. Burns, regardless of their source, kill or maim several thousands each year. Considerable research is being conducted to help treat the burned patient. Today individuals have a better chance of surviving after receiving severe burns, but must face a long recovery period during which infection and shock must be fought, and plastic surgery endured.

HEAT EXHAUSTION

Heat exhaustion (also called heat prostration) is caused by prolonged exposure to excessive heat, particularly in combination with high humidity. As the temperature increases, blood accumulates in the skin, and perspiration increases in an effort to cool the body. Consequently less blood is available for circulation and the blood supply to the brain is diminished. As this condition progresses, fainting may result due to the lack of oxygen available to the brain. Individuals most susceptible to heat exhaustion include the elderly, alcoholics, persons with circulatory problems, the overweight, and those unaccustomed to working or exercising in hot, humid environments. Women tend to be more susceptible to heat exhaustion than men.

Indicators of Heat Exhaustion

In mild cases of heat exhaustion the individual may feel fatigued, nauseated, and faint. The skin may become pale and clammy and he may complain of headache. As the condition progresses, the individual perspires profusely and his pulse is rapid but weak. The pupils may become dilated, breathing is shallow, and vomiting may occur. In rare instances an individual may lapse into unconsciousness. It is important that the first aider be able to differentiate the indicators for heat exhaustion from those for heat stroke, which is far more serious and presents a more life-threatening situation.

First Aid Procedures for Heat Exhaustion

The individual should be made as comfortable as possible by loosening any tight clothing and having him lie down. He should be encouraged to take fluids and if his pulse is very weak, stimulants such as cool black coffee or tea may be given. Salt tablets or a salt solution (one-half teaspoon salt in a half glass of water) may be taken by mouth to replenish the salt lost through heavy perspiration. In some instances oxygen may be administered if available. As the individual recovers, do not allow him to become overly active until he has rested for a period of time.

HEAT STROKE

The normal body temperature is 98.6 degrees Fahrenheit. When the external atmosphere is hot, perspiration increases so as to cool the body and maintain its normal temperature. When the body's heat-regulating mechanism fails, perspiration decreases or ceases completely, causing the body temperature to rise. If body temperature continues to rise unchecked, the high fever will cause serious damage to such vital organs as the kidneys or brain. Unless recognized and treated immediately, heat stroke may be fatal.

Unlike heat exhaustion, heat stroke affects men more often than women. It is also more common among the middle-aged and elderly and heavy users of alcohol. It is caused by exposure to high temperatures especially where humidity is high and air circulation poor. Persons exerting themselves physically in this type of environment are more likely candidates for heat stroke.

Indicators of Heat Stroke

In the early stages of heat stroke, the individual's skin will feel noticeably hot and dry, and appear flushed. His pulse will be rapid and breathing will be deep. As the condition progresses, body temperature will rapidly rise to as high as 108 degrees or even higher. If the body remains at these temperatures for any period of time, brain and kidney tissue begin to coagulate. The individual's pulse now becomes weak and thready, and respiration becomes shallow. Muscle twitching may change to convulsions. Pupils of the eye become dilated, and an offensive body odor is present. Skin color will turn ashen gray, an indication that the individual is in or near cardiovascular collapse.

First Aid Procedures for Heat Stroke

Since heat stroke is a very grave condition, positive steps to lower body temperature must be taken immediately. Body temperature may be reduced in a number of ways:

1. Move the victim to a cool environment immediately.
2. Loosen or remove tight clothing.
3. Douse the body with cold water or sponge with rubbing alcohol. Ideally, submerge the victim in a tub of cold water containing ice.
4. Check and care for shock.

[108]   Burns and Exposure

If available, oxygen may be administered. A salt solution, as described in heat exhaustion, may be given to conscious individuals.

Heat stroke is a serious emergency and quick action is necessary if death is to be prevented. While the first aider is taking action to reduce body temperature, someone should be calling an ambulance to transport the individual to a medical facility.

HEAT CRAMPS

Heat cramps are caused by prolonged physical exertion in high temperatures. Usually, the victim has lost large quantities of body salt due to excessive perspiration. This is especially true of persons who drink large quantities of water and are physically active in environments of high temperatures.

Indicators of Heat Cramps

The individual will complain of severe cramps in the abdomen or in the muscles of the lower limbs. These cramps may be very painful if salt depletion is extreme. The individual is extremely thirsty, and may feel dizzy, nauseated. His pulse will be strong and rapid; body temperature is usually normal or slightly elevated. Skin color is pale and perspiration is excessive. In extreme cases the individual may become unconscious.

First Aid Procedures for Heat Cramps

The person suffering from heat cramps should cease physical activity and rest in a cool environment. Body salt should be replenished by giving a salt solution or salt tablets as for heat exhaustion. Application of pressure or moist warm towels directly over the affected area will help relax the cramped muscles and lessen pain. Preventive measures are most effective for heat cramps. If one expects to be physically active in a hot environment for any length of time, he should take salt tablets or a salt solution three or four times during the day.

BURNS (1) (2) (3) (4)

Burns are classified according to their source, extent, and depth. There are various sources of burns: (1) thermal (hot gasses, solids, liquids, or friction); (2) corrosive (strong chemicals such as acids and alkalies); (3) electrical (either manufactured or natural electricity); and (4) radiation sources such as ultraviolet rays or atomic radiation. In general, the length

Burns and Exposure   [109]

of time the individual is exposed to the heat source will determine how severely he will be injured. For example, if you touch your finger to a hot iron for just a split second a minor burn results, but if contact lasts for any length of time, a deep serious burn will develop.

Indicators of Burns

The extent to which the individual is burned is probably the greatest single variable in determining the seriousness of the burn and chances for recovery. An individual with deep (third degree) burns covering 50 to 80 percent of the body surface is not likely to survive, but the younger the individual, the better his chances. Individuals with less serious (second degree) burns covering 20 to 70 percent of the body surface can usually be saved with prompt medical attention. Minor (first degree) burns covering 10 to 20 percent of the body surface require medical attention, but usually do not present a life-threatening situation. In order to estimate how extensive the burns are, the "Rule of Nine" has been devised (Figure 7.1). By knowing what percentage of the body surface

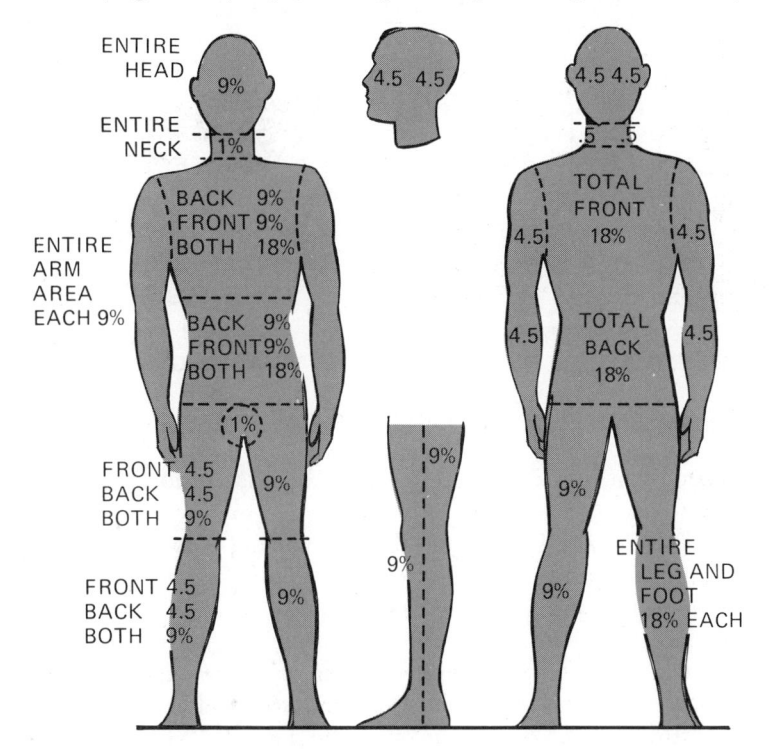

Figure 7.1 Rule of Nine for estimating percent of body surface burned in an adult.

[110] Burns and Exposure

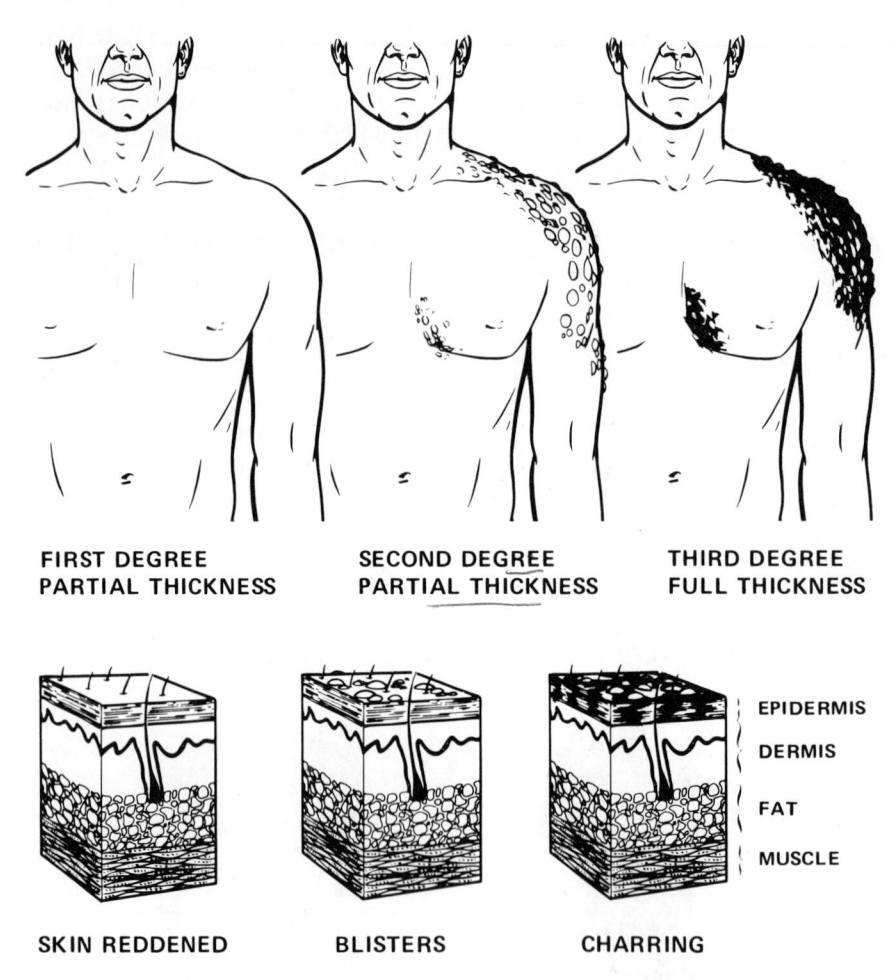

| FIRST DEGREE | SECOND DEGREE | THIRD DEGREE |
| PARTIAL THICKNESS | PARTIAL THICKNESS | FULL THICKNESS |

SKIN REDDENED — BLISTERS — CHARRING

EPIDERMIS
DERMIS
FAT
MUSCLE

Figure 7.2 Classification of burns according to skin depth damaged.

is involved, one can quickly determine the potential seriousness of the injury.

All burns, even minor first-degree burns involving 9 to 10 percent of the body surface, require medical attention. A burn is an open wound, and the danger of infection is always present.

The third factor in determining the seriousness of a burn is the depth of the burn. Classification according to layer of skin damage is shown in Figure 7.2. *First-degree burns,* such as sunburn, scalds, and scorches from irons or stoves, involve only the outer (epidermal) layer of skin. The skin turns red and the affected area is usually quite painful because the sensory nerve endings may be exposed to air or slightly injured. *Second-*

degree burns are characterized by blisters. The heat source has now penetrated deeper and interstitual fluid is accumulating between the layers of skin. Shock and pain are often complicators in this burn. *Third-degree burns* are the most serious, involving deep tissue destruction. Affected areas may be burned so severely as to appear charred, with portions of tissue missing, bones exposed or even destroyed. Pain is not usually a complicator because the nerve endings have been destroyed. Shock and infection, however, may prove to be life-threatening. In general an individual who is severely burned is likely to sustain a combination of first-, second-, and third-degree burns. The inner deepest portion of the burn will be the most serious (third degree) and the degree of seriousness will lessen as you move away from the center (Figure 7.3). Initially, the depth may not be apparent in a burn until the outer layer of skin has been removed to expose a much deeper wound. First- and second-degree burns can heal on their own, but third-degree burns require supportive grafting treatment in order to heal.

Another possible complication in severe burns, particularly burns about the face and upper body, is the inhalation of superheated air. This causes the respiratory tract and lungs to become burned and often proves fatal.

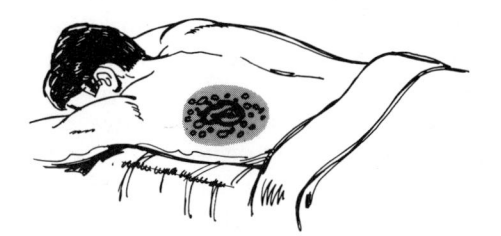

Figure 7.3 Radiating effect seen with serious burns.

First Aid Procedures for Burns

Although burn cases may be serious, they usually do not present the same immediate life-threatening risk as do severe hemorrhage, respiratory failure, and cardiac arrest. The first aider does not treat the burn itself, but renders valuable assistance in making the victim more comfortable and facilitating subsequent treatment by medical personnel. Traditional methods of applying butter or various ointments only hamper treatment and may introduce infection.

Regardless of the degree of seriousness, the three objectives to keep in mind with all burns are: (1) prevent contamination, (2) prevent shock, and (3) relieve pain. If these three objectives can be accomplished, the burned individual will have improved chances of recovery. Contamination is prevented by carefully exposing the burned area and covering it with as large a sterile dressing as is necessary. Special care must be taken not to pull clothing from a burn, but rather to cut the clothing around the burn to expose it. If a large portion of the body is involved, it is advisable to wrap the entire body in a sterile sheet or cloth. To prevent shock it is important to keep the victim lying flat, administer fluids (if he is conscious), and conserve body heat. The first aider may help relieve pain by simply covering the exposed wound. This is particularly true of first- and second-degree burns, where the sensory nerve endings are exposed or injured. Do not administer any aspirin or similar pain-killing drug. A first aider must remember to accomplish all three of these objectives in all burn cases, regardless of the seriousness of the burn. In addition, procedures helpful in caring for particular kinds of burns are described below.

First-Degree Burns

Although first-degree burns are the least severe and will heal on their own, the first aider can initiate therapy to relieve pain and promote healing. Research and practice have shown that applications of cold water are helpful. If possible, immerse the affected area in cold water containing shaved ice, or apply cold water packs to the affected area. The cold water seems to help in removing heat from the body, serves as a mild local anesthetic to relieve pain, and may prevent further tissue destruction. If cold water is applied immediately, the depth of the burn may be lessened considerably. For example, a potential second-degree burn may be turned into a first-degree burn if cold is applied quickly enough. Some doctors also recommend the use of a mild local analgesic such as Solarcaine, but it is best to check with a physician before using such products. When greasy creams, ointments, or butter are used, infection may be introduced, the burn becomes masked, and it may take considerable time and cause pain to remove these products before the physician can properly treat the burn.

Second-Degree Burns

Cold water may also be used on second-degree burns. One must be very careful not to open any blisters which have formed. The physician may elect to remove the outer layer of skin, or leave it as its own dressing. Either way, the first aider should only cover the affected area or use a mild, recommended anesthetic and seek medical attention. In making the burned individual comfortable, it is wise to loosen or remove any constricting clothing or jewelry, to prevent complications in case swelling occurs.

Third-Degree Burns

For third-degree burns there is little to be done by a first aider. The burn should be exposed (as previously discussed) and covered with a sterile dressing, and medical attention should be sought immediately. Shock and infection are possible, and everything must be done to prevent these conditions from developing.

Inhalation of Superheated Air

If an individual is burned about the face and upper portion of the body, he may have inhaled superheated air. In this case the first aider must assume that the respiratory tract and lungs have also been burned along with any visible outer burns. The individual may complain of a sore throat or hoarseness, or he may be coughing and having difficulty breathing. Nasal hair may be singed and the nose swollen and red. The first aider can do little more than observe the individual carefully for respiratory difficulty, maintain an open airway, and seek medical attention immediately. Oxygen, if available, may be administered. Burns of the lungs and respiratory tract are often fatal, especially if pulmonary edema develops.

Electrical and Chemical Burns

An individual may receive an electrical burn from direct contact with an electrical wire or by being struck by lightening. The burns received as the current enters and exits from the body vary, and may not be immediately apparent to the first aider. Of more immediate concern is the effect of the electricity upon the respiratory and circulatory systems. High voltage burns can be quite extensive, particularly internally. The external burns should be treated as third-degree burns, as previously discussed.

Chemical burns result when an individual comes in direct contact with a strong corrosive substance such as an acid or alkali. When neutralizing or counteracting agents are administered they may inflict further damage because they may (1) be too strong and additionally burn the individual; (2) produce heat in the reaction with the corrosive and further burn the individual; or (3) produce a salt which itself is damaging to the individual. Therefore instead of attempting to neutralize the chemical, it is recommended that the first aider remove any contaminated clothing and dilute the burning chemical with large quantities of water. Continue to flush the area for a period of time and seek medical attention. Chemical burns of the eyes are particularly dangerous as the eye is easily damaged. The eyes should be flushed with flowing water as illustrated in Figure

[114] Burns and Exposure

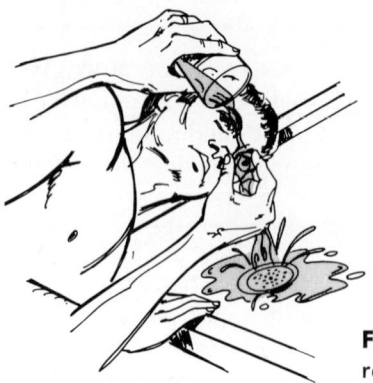

Figure 7.4 Flushing the eye with water to remove chemicals or foreign matter.

7.4. Acids tend to burn immediately and are easily flushed out, whereas alkalies tend to penetrate deeper and take longer to burn, so continuous flushing is particularly important in the case of alkaline burns.

Sunburn

During exposure to the sun the ultraviolet rays are absorbed by the body and produce changes under the skin which lead to the much sought-after suntan. Long exposure to direct ultraviolet rays, however, may cause first- or second-degree burns. Cancer researchers are also finding that prolonged exposure (15 to 20 years) to ultraviolet rays may cause skin cancer. Most susceptible are farmers, ranchers, ship employees, and those who work constantly out in the open. Sunburn is basically a first- or second-degree burn and should be treated as any other first- or second-degree burn. Nausea, infection, and possibly sun-poisoning may occur in severe cases of sunburn. Medical attention should be sought if over 10 percent of the body surface is involved. Prevention, of course, is the key, and fair-skinned individuals need to be especially precautious. Besides, an even tanning built up gradually by increasing periods of exposure is more cosmetic and longer lasting.

ADVERSE EFFECTS OF COLD

Just as the body is affected by extremes in the upper temperature ranges, so it can be affected by extremes in the lower temperature ranges, that is to say by cold and direct contact with cold liquids. The probability of general cooling or frostbite are influenced not only by cold temperatures but also by the humidity and the wind-chill factor (see Figure 7.5).

Figure 7.5 INDEX OF WIND-CHILL FACTOR

Wind	Degrees Fahrenheit Dry-Bulb Temperature														
	35	30	25	20	15	10	5	0	−5	−10	−15	−20	−25	−30
	Equivalent Degrees														
Calm	35	30	25	20	15	10	5	0	−5	−10	−15	−20	−25	−30
5 mph	33	27	21	16	12	7	1	−6	−11	−15	−20	−26	−31	−35
10 mph	21	16	9	2	−2	−9	−15	−22	−27	−31	−38	−45	−52	−58
15 mph	16	11	1	−6	−11	−18	−25	−33	−40	−45	−51	−60	−65	−70
20 mph	12	3	−4	−9	−17	−24	−32	−40	−46	−52	−60	−68	−76	−81
25 mph	7	0	−7	−15	−22	−29	−37	−45	−52	−58	−67	−75	−83	−89
30 mph	5	−2	−11	−18	−26	−33	−41	−49	−56	−63	−70	−78	−87	−94
35 mph	3	−4	−13	−20	−27	−35	−43	−52	−60	−67	−72	−83	−90	−98
40 mph	1	−4	−15	−22	−29	−36	−45	−54	−62	−69	−76	−87	−94	−101

COLD · VERY COLD · BITTER COLD · EXTREME COLD

This chart shows how the cooling power of different temperatures varies under various wind conditions. For example, under calm conditions, a temperature of 15°F has a cooling power of 15°, but if it is accompanied by a ten mile an hour wind, it has a cooling power equivalent to −2°F. (From *Emergency Care and Transportation of the Sick and Injured*, American Academy of Orthopaedic Surgeons, Chicago, Ill., 1971. Used with permission.)

[116] Burns and Exposure

Frostbite

Frostbite occurs when portions of the body are subjected to cold causing local injury or tissue destruction. Areas of the body most commonly affected by frostbite are the toes, ears, nose, and fingers, because these areas are at the end of a circulatory route or have a limited normal blood supply. When an individual is subjected to a cold environment or a cold liquid, the body attempts to circulate warmth-giving blood to all tissues. As the temperature drops, the peripheral circulatory system begins to constrict (as in shock) in order to protect the vital internal organs. The tissue is then further endangered as not enough warmth is present to prevent freezing. An individual's tolerance to cold varies. Figure 7.6 illustrates how quickly the body will freeze at various temperatures. Frostbite is a greater hazard for individuals who are elderly, have a dark-pigmented skin, or are in poor physical condition. Fatigue, nervousness, impaired circulation, or alcohol further increase vulnerability. In addi-

Figure 7.6 FREEZING TIME FOR THE BODY

Time	Wind Velocity	Temperature F.
Less than one minute	20 mph	32 below
	30 mph	25 below
	40 mph	20 below
Less than two minutes	10 mph	37 below
	20 mph	27 below
	30 mph	17 below
	40 mph	15 below
5 minutes	10 mph	36 below
	20 mph	20 below
	30 mph	12 below
	40 mph	6 below
15 minutes	10 mph	16 below
	20 mph	5 below
	30 mph	1 above
	40 mph	5 above
25 minutes	10 mph	17 below
	20 mph	5 below
	30 mph	1 above
	40 mph	5 above
60 minutes	10 mph	1 above
	20 mph	12 above
	30 mph	16 above
	40 mph	20 above

From O. C. Kreymborg, M.D., "First Aid," *Fire Chief Magazine*, February 1971.

tion, individuals who have previously suffered from exposure or frostbite seem to be more susceptible.

Indicators of Frostbite

Prior to actual freezing of the tissues, the body warning system is activated. This warning system involves a tingling sensation and gradual numbness. Initially the affected area may become painful and the skin turns violet-red in color. Additionally, burning and itching usually occur. Unless the individual is removed from the cold environment at this point, severe freezing may ensue. As cold exposure continues, the skin turns a dead-white or grayish-yellow and ice crystals form internally. Eventually a complete loss of sensation occurs. Some individuals may not realize this is occurring to them and may have to be told and rather strongly urged to move into a warmer environment. If not treated, severe frostbite may develop into gangrene with amputation being the only alternative to death.

First Aid Procedures for Frostbite

There are many theories as to the best treatment of frostbite. Some advocate rubbing the affected area with snow or ice; others advocate gradual re-warming. Rubbing the affected part of the body in snow or ice is quite harmful as it only serves to increase the extent of damage by applying more cold. Slow re-warming at room temperature is a long and painful process and may lead to eventual tissue destruction. Physicians are now recommending a rapid re-warming process which helps to eliminate further tissue destruction.

Not only is it important to begin re-warming the frozen part, but it is vitally important to remove the individual from the cold environment. During movement into a warmer environment, attempt to protect the affected area from further injury and wrap it in warm blankets or woolen clothing. Once the individual is in a warmer area, a more rapid re-warming may be begun. If at all possible the affected part should be immersed in warm, not hot, water. Temperatures between 103 and 107 degrees Fahrenheit seem to be most desirable. Remove any constricting clothing such as boots, socks, and gloves, but do not allow the individual to walk or support his own weight if the feet are affected. Warm stimulating liquids such as tea, coffee, or soup may be given to the victim. During the freezing process ice crystals have formed. Rubbing in an attempt to re-warm the affected area is quite harmful as these crystals act like splinters and may cause tissue damage. During the thawing process the skin becomes red and swollen, and large blisters may form. Do not attempt to open these blisters. Do not let the individual smoke, because nicotine causes vasoconstriction which is opposite of what is desired for re-warming. As the affected portion is re-warmed, encourage mild exercise or use of the area to increase circulation. The affected area should be covered with a sterile dressing. While transporting the individual to a medical facility, observe closely for shock. The ultimate tissue damage may not be known until a period of medical observation has taken place.

Generalized Cooling

At times, the entire body is suffering from overexposure to cold, for example, from near drowning or being lost in the woods. Local freezing (frostbite) may occur, but exposure is apparent over the entire body. This individual feels cold, is shivering, and must be brought into a warmer environment as quickly as possible. Wrap in warm blankets and give hot liquids such as tea, soup, or coffee. Do not give alcoholic beverages. Otherwise treat as previously discussed for local frostbite.

{ 8 }
POISONINGS

Approximately 3,000 individuals die annually as a result of poisoning or overdose by drugs, chemicals, gases, or foods. In addition, over half a million children, the majority under age five, accidentally ingest a sufficient amount of a toxic product or combination of products to require medical attention. Poisons may cause different reactions in the body depending upon the individual, the amount of poison taken, and the poison itself. An increasing number of individuals are being affected either by deliberate ingestion of a harmful substance or by accidental overdose. Regardless of the individual's intent, the first aider must work quickly in order to minimize the amount of bodily harm and, in some instance, to prevent death. Just as severe hemorrhage and respiratory and circulatory failure are considered life-threatening, so must we consider an instance of poisoning or overdose, until proven that the amount taken was not lethal.

POISON CONTROL CENTERS

In 1953, the Chicago chapter of the American Academy of Pediatrics formed the first poison control center. Physicians in the area were concerned about the growing numbers of children who accidentally ingested a household product containing a harmful substance. As new products came on the market with new chemical formulas, it was becoming increasingly difficult for each individual physician to keep up to date and to prescribe the correct medical treatment called for. So in order to assist physicians in identifying poisons and treating children, the first poison control center was formed. As the program grew (there were 16 centers by 1957), the centers developed three objectives:

1. To collect data on the toxicity of products and on medical treatment.
2. To compile statistics.
3. To develop poison prevention program for the general public.

Originally the centers were established for use by physicians only. Today there are over 520 centers throughout the United States operating 24 hours a day, usually staffed by volunteers, with medical advice close by. Most poison control centers accept calls from the lay public, but a few restrict participation to medical personnel. First aiders and others should check with their local center to determine the policy in their area.

When an individual has swallowed a poison or taken a substance suspected of containing poison, the nearest poison control center should be phoned at once. The caller should report the name of the product, the quantity taken, and the age and approximate weight of the individual. The center will then check its product information records (sample labels are also filed) and issue the following advice: (a) the product is poisonous and harmful in the amount ingested, therefore seek medical attention immediately; or (b) there is no immediate danger, but consultation with your family physician is recommended; or (c) the product is harmless, but watch for any other signs. In addition, if the product *is* poisonous the center also instructs the caller whether to induce emesis, dilute, or give an antidote prior to transporting the individual to a hospital.

The National Clearing House for Poison Control Centers, Washington, D.C., under the Department of Health, Education, and Welfare, is responsible for keeping each center supplied with the latest information on all products and treatment. They work closely with manufacturers and may consult with them directly when the need arises. The statistics kept by each center are forwarded to the National Clearing House where they are compiled and made available to the public along with information on safety and prevention. Data collected for 1973 indicate that 44.3% of poison incidents were from medicines (aspirin accounted for 6.6%); 16.3% from petroleum products; 8.8% from pesticides; 8.4% from cleaning and polishing agents; 6.0% from turpentine and paints; 4.8% from gases and vapors; 4.2% from cosmetics; 0.1% from plants; and 9.6% miscellaneous. Manufacturers are required by the Food and Drug Administration to show prominently on the label that the product may be harmful, or, if poisonous, to indicate the antidote. Despite all precautions, however, accidents continue to happen. Prevention is still the key to control, which means that everyone must be made aware of the dangers and should be instructed in the proper use, storage, and disposal of potentially harmful products.

POISON ENTRY ROUTES

Poisonous substances enter the body in four ways. *Ingestion,* or swallowing, is probably the most common, especially with children and in incidents of overdose. *Inhalation* is the entrance through the respiratory system, for example, by breathing in noxious fumes. *Injection* involves direct entrance into the bloodstream through the capillaries, arteries, or veins. Examples include snake bites and insect bites, or hypodermic injections. *Absorption* through the skin is the fourth mode of entry. This occurs with pesticide and herbicide sprays and poisonous contact plants such as ivy, oak, and sumac.

Once the toxic product is within the body it reacts in various manners. The tissue may be burned or destroyed through contact with corrosive chemicals such as strong acids and alkalies. The central nervous system may be either extremely depressed (as with barbiturates, morphine, or alcohol) or severely stimulated (as with insecticides or strychnine) causing respiratory failures or convulsions. The poison may also replace the oxygen needed for survival, as in carbon monoxide poisoning. Regardless of the ultimate damage, the first aider must act quickly to prevent even greater damage from occurring.

INGESTED POISONS

When poisoning is suspected, there are specific ways to help determine what poison has been ingested. If the individual is conscious, talk with him and try to find out what he has swallowed. Look around carefully (but quickly) for any empty or open bottles or other containers, especially in the kitchen, bedroom, and bathroom. (Any containers you find should be taken to the hospital.) Observe the individual for burns and stains, especially about the mouth and on the fingers, or a peculiar odor on the breath. These are usually indicators that a corrosive poison has been ingested, and will require special emergency procedures and treatment. In other cases, the individual may be complaining of abdominal pain and nausea. Further, if a depressant drug has been taken, the individual may appear sluggish or drowsy, or may be having difficulty breath-

Figure 8.1   POISON DECISION CHART

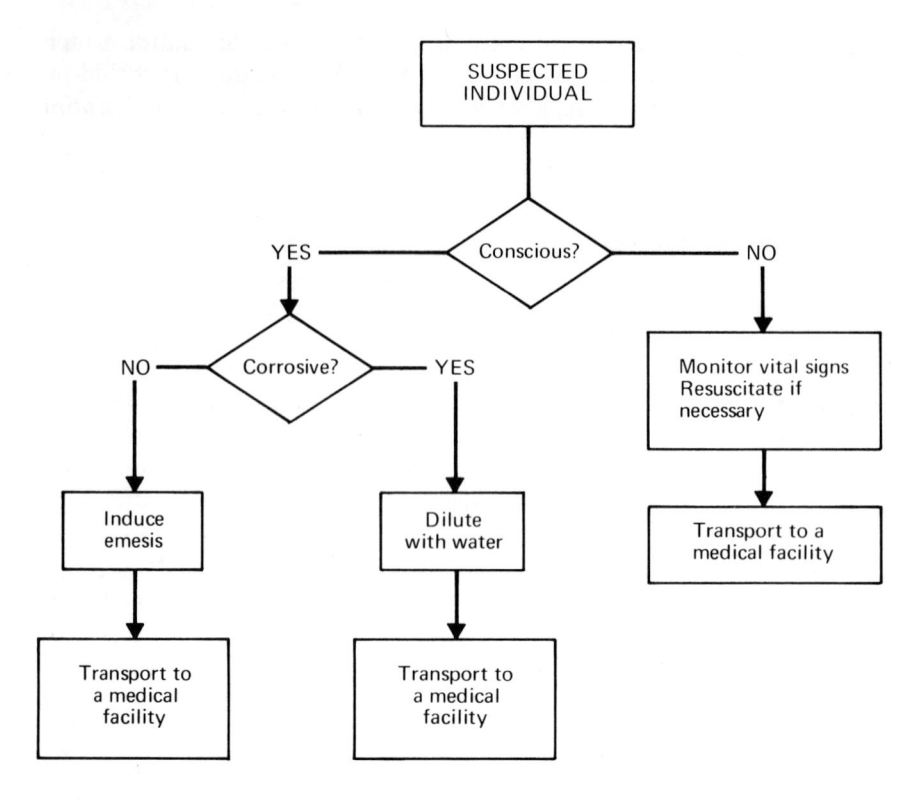

```
                    SUSPECTED
                    INDIVIDUAL
                         │
                         ▼
          YES ──── Conscious? ──── NO
           │                        │
           ▼                        ▼
   NO ── Corrosive? ── YES    ┌──────────────┐
    │                │        │ Monitor vital signs
    │                │        │ Resuscitate if
    │                │        │ necessary
    ▼                ▼        └──────────────┘
 ┌────────┐     ┌────────┐            │
 │ Induce │     │ Dilute │            ▼
 │ emesis │     │ with   │     ┌──────────────┐
 └────────┘     │ water  │     │ Transport to a│
     │          └────────┘     │ medical facility│
     ▼              │          └──────────────┘
 ┌────────┐         ▼
 │Transport│    ┌────────┐
 │to a     │    │Transport│
 │medical  │    │to a     │
 │facility │    │medical  │
 └────────┘     │facility │
                └────────┘
```

NOTE: If uncertain whether the poison is corrosive or noncorrosive, call the nearest Poison Control Center for advice.

ing. If the individual is unconscious, look around for open bottles; observe him for burns, stains, and mouth odor; and watch particularly for any respiratory and circulatory difficulty. Once you have determined (a) whether or not the poison ingested is corrosive, and (b) whether or not the victim is still conscious, first aid care may begin (Figure 8.1).

Corrosive Poisons

When burns or stains appear about the mouth, fingers, or lips, or there is a peculiar odor on the breath (something like kerosene, ammonia, or Lysol), or if the label on the container shows that the product contains either acid or alkali, *do not induce vomiting.* Products containing acids or alkalis corrode, burn, or eat away tissue, especially the mucous membranes, as they enter the body. In addition to their immediate corrosive action, they cause inflammation of the deeper tissues and in some instances produce harmful effects through the absorption process. If vomiting occurs, additional corrosion results while the product is leaving the body; fumes may be inhaled causing a chemical pneumonia condition in the lungs; vomitus may enter the thoracic cavity through the perforated tissues.

The most common corrosive chemicals are the strong acids and alkalies listed below, which are used as cleaning agents, solvents, and disinfectants either in pure form or in commercial compounds.

Corrosive Acids	Corrosive Alkalies
Hydrochloric acid (metal cleaners)	Potash or caustic potash (drain cleaners)
Sulfuric acid (auto batteries)	
Nitric acid (industrial cleaning solutions)	Caustic soda or lye (soap-making)
Oxalic acid (cleaning agent)	Unslaked lime (building trades)
Carbolic acid (disinfectants such as Lysol)	Ammonia water (cleaning agent)

If an individual has ingested a corrosive product and is conscious, begin by getting him to drink a glass of plain water to immediately dilute the corrosive. Getting the victim to drink water may not be easy because the mouth and esophagus may be burned, making it painful to swallow, but the first aider should try his best to get him to drink. The amount of water will vary with the individual, but it should never be so much as to distend the stomach and induce vomiting unintentionally. If the specific corrosive is known, a neutralizer may be given if available. An effective neutralizer for a corrosive acid would be limewater, chalk and water, small amounts of diluted milk of magnesia, or a teaspoon of baking soda dissolved in water. To counteract a corrosive alkali, give large amounts of lemon or other citrus juice or a mixture of water and vinegar in equal parts. The individual should be checked and cared for shock, which is common in corrosive poisoning, and transported to a medical facility as soon as possible. Time should not be lost in trying to find a neutralizer as this will be available at the hospital.

If the individual is found unconscious, maintain an open airway, observe for vomiting, care for shock, and seek medical attention immediately.

Petroleum Distillates

Petroleum distillates are found in furniture polishes, lighter fluids, kerosene, gasoline, insecticide sprays, and various other commercial compounds. Poisoning may occur by ingestion or by inhalation of these substances. The victim may choke, cough, gasp, appear to be strangling, or may begin vomiting upon ingestion. A strong odor of the product will usually be present. Do not attempt to induce emesis, but rather dilute with water and seek medical attention. If the individual—particularly if a child—begins to vomit on his own, prevent him from aspirating vomited matter or from taking the fumes back into the lungs. Place the individual on his side with the head lower than the rest of the body during transport to a medical facility.

Noncorrosive Poisons

If the poison ingested is not a corrosive, then the procedure is aimed at getting it out of the body as fast as possible. For the longer the poison remains in the stomach the greater the risk of its being absorbed into the circulatory system and resulting in permanent damage, even death. If the individual is conscious, get him to drink a couple of glasses of water to dilute the poison, and then induce vomiting. Vomiting may be induced by tickling the back of the throat or by giving an emetic such as soapy water, dry mustard and water, or salt and water. It is often difficult to get an individual, particularly a child, to swallow any of these mixtures. Better luck may be had with syrup of ipecac, a commercial emetic sold without a prescription in one-ounce containers. This is a thick, sweet, cherry-flavored liquid which induces emesis rather effortlessly. One-half ounce (one tablespoon) taken with a couple of glasses of water usually induces vomiting in ten to twenty minutes. If vomiting does not occur, the second half-ounce is administered. (A sample of the vomitus should be retained for laboratory analysis.) An antidote or counteractant may now be administered. This may be either the specific antidote recommended on the product label or the universal antidote sold in most pharmacies under the name Unidote, which is taken with a glass of water. After the antidote has been allowed to remain in the stomach for three or four minutes, induce emesis once again, and continue the process until the vomitus is clear. Once the stomach has been emptied, a soothing substance (known as a "demulcent") such as milk, egg white, or olive oil may be given to coat the stomach lining. During this entire procedure the individual should be checked and cared for shock, and the care should continue while he is being transported to a hospital. In most cases the individual will vomit while en route to the hospital or upon arrival, so that it is usually not necessary for the first aider to proceed beyond inducing emesis.

If the individual is found unconscious, none of the procedures described above should be followed. The only action indicated for the first aider is to maintain an open airway, check and care for shock, and seek immediate medical attention.

Barbiturate Poisoning

When taken in the proper dosages, sedative drugs (barbiturates) are relatively safe, but in overdoses they may prove fatal. In fact such drugs are the most common method of attempted suicide. Barbiturates are used to depress the central nervous system and generally promote sleep. Taken in combination with alcohol, which is also a central nervous system depressant, the effects are heightened and death may ensue in a very short period of time.

If the individual is found conscious, he may appear to be drowsy, mentally confused, and may be suffering from hallucinations. His speech may be slurred, the pulse weak, and breathing shallow. Emesis should be induced by whatever means possible and continued so as to empty the stomach of as much barbiturate as possible. Drinking strong coffee and walking about are not particularly helpful. Administer oxygen if available and transport to a medical facility as soon as possible.

If the individual is found unconscious, observe his breathing and circulation carefully. Unconsciousness usually indicates that the barbiturate has entered the circulatory system in sufficient quantities to affect the brain. Maintain an open airway and administer oxygen if available. Cardiopulmonary resuscitation may be necessary in severe cases. Care for shock and transport to a medical facility immediately.

Salicylate Poisoning

Salicylate poisoning occurs most often as a result of an overdose of aspirin. The quantity of aspirin necessary to produce symptoms is difficult to determine. It depends upon the age, weight, and general condition of the individual involved. Infants and young children are more susceptible than adults. The symptoms of overdose may not develop for 12 to 24 hours following ingestion, and in accumulative doses it may take one to four days before the symptoms appear. Usually the first and most dependable sign is rapid, deep breathing with no known explanation. If allowed to continue unchecked, this may lead to adverse body chemistry changes. The clotting time of the blood is affected and stomach hemorrhage is not uncommon. If vomiting occurs it is the color of coffee grounds. A skin rash and bleeding from the gums and mucous membranes may also occur. The individual will be irritable and restless or may convulse and become semi-conscious; he may complain of ringing in the ears and dizziness, and may experience acute abdominal pain, fever, and delirium. Not all these symptoms appear in all individuals; some are more common in children while others appear more often in adults. Any combination of the above symptoms, however, should be suspect and action should be taken accordingly.

If the individual has just swallowed a quantity of aspirin, emesis will be of value, but if 12 to 24 hours have elapsed since ingestion, emesis will

Figure 8.2 COMMON FOOD POISONINGS

Type and Cause	Reaction	Food Source	Onset	Indicators	First Aid Measures
Amanita phalloides	Liquifies tissues, especially red blood cells; 50% fatal	A poisonous wild mushroom	6 to 24 hours	Acute abdominal pain; diarrhea; vomiting; periods of recovery; shock; convulsions; coma	Emesis if necessary; care for shock; medical attention
Amanita muscaria Muscarine, a highly toxic substance	Affects the nervous system; often fatal	A poisonous wild mushroom (common name "fly agaric") with orange cap and white gills	A few minutes to three hours	Violent vomiting; diarrhea; a flow of tears; excessive saliva; profuse sweating; difficult breathing	Bed rest; emesis if necessary; care for shock; medical attention
Shellfish Bacterial contamination due to improper refrigeration or storage	Acute gastroenteritis	Crabs, shrimp, lobster, clams, mussels, oysters, snails, etc.; raw or cooked seafood dishes	Usually within half an hour	Violent intestinal upset; generalized blotchy red-blue rash with severe itching; generalized swelling; convulsions; wheezing	Maintain open airway; immediate medical attention
Staphylococcal Bacterial action due to improper refrigeration or storage	Violent intestinal upset; often called intestinal grippe	All kinds of meats, especially cold cuts; dairy products; baked goods containing creams and custards; foods containing mayonnaise	2 to 6 hours	Nausea; vomiting; abdominal pain; diarrhea; weakness; often headaches; muscular pain; collapse	No specific treatment; will recover after toxin leaves body by vomiting and diarrhea

Salmonella Bacterial action due to contamination	Acute gastroenteritis	Greatest single source is poultry products; also meats, dairy products, and vegetables	8 or more hours	Nausea; vomiting; abdominal pain; watery diarrhea; chills followed by fever to 102° F.	No specific treatment; seek medical attention for correction of dehydration; antibiotics available
Botulism Bacterial action	Affects the motor nerve system; 75% fatal if untreated; death due to strangulation or cardiac failure	Improperly canned or preserved foods	4 to 48 hours or longer	Disturbed vision; dimness, double vision; paralysis of eye muscles; difficulty in swallowing, talking, and breathing; incoordination; paralysis of throat muscles	Get prompt medical attention for administration of antitoxin.
Trichinosis Parasitic round-worm	Affects muscle tissues	Insufficiently cooked pork from infested hogs	2 to 28 days	Backache; headache; high fever; muscle pain; stomach cramps; general weakness; chills	Seek medical attention immediately

be ineffective. In the latter instance, maintain an open airway and transport to a medical facility as rapidly as possible.

Food Poisoning

Certain bacteria and chemicals in foods or utilized during handling and preparation may produce adverse effects upon the body. Food poisoning does not generally prove fatal in itself, but may lead to changes within the body which, when complicated by old age, poor physical condition, or chronic illnesses, may produce death. Figure 8.2 is a chart of the more common types of food poisons, their effects, indicators, and the first aid procedures to be followed.

Summary of Procedures for Ingested Poisons

To provide the first aider with a handy reference guide, we reprint in Figure 8.3 a chart prepared by *American Druggist*, giving the explicit procedure to follow when certain poisons or overdoses are ingested. Whenever there is doubt about the product's toxicity and whether to induce emesis, call the nearest poison control center for advice.

INHALED POISONS

Poisons can enter the body readily through the respiratory system. Two dangerous gases often inhaled are carbon monoxide and chlorine. Carbon monoxide is a by-product of combustion; chlorine is used extensively in purification of water, especially swimming pools. Other gases which produce harmful effects upon the body when inhaled are used primarily in industry and by highly specialized professions, and are not generally available to the public. When accidents involving these specialized chemicals occur, the injured individual is transported rapidly to a medical facility for assistance. There is little a first aider may do to assist these individuals, as oxygen and specialized medical care are required.

Carbon Monoxide

Carbon monoxide is a colorless, tasteless, odorless gas given off during combustion. It may be found in automobile exhaust, illuminating gas, sewer gas, smoke, stoves, and heaters. Since it is so undetectable, poisoning may occur in minutes if the concentration is high in an unventilated area. Death is caused because the carbon monoxide molecule unites with hemoglobin of the red blood cells more readily than oxygen, preventing the formation of oxyhemoglobin which is required for life. Even rela-

Figure 8.3

Poison Antidote and Drug Counterdose Chart

DO THIS FIRST

- Send for a doctor—immediately.
- Keep the patient warm.
- Determine if the patient has taken
  (1) A POISON
  (2) AN OVERDOSE
- While waiting for physician, give appropriate counterdose below.
- But do not force any liquids on the patient — if he is unconscious.

- And do not induce vomiting if patient is having convulsions.

To Find The Correct Counterdose
- In one of the lists printed at right, find substance causing the trouble.
- Next to that substance is a number. This refers to counterdose bearing same number in the section below.

Keep all poisons and medicines out of reach of children

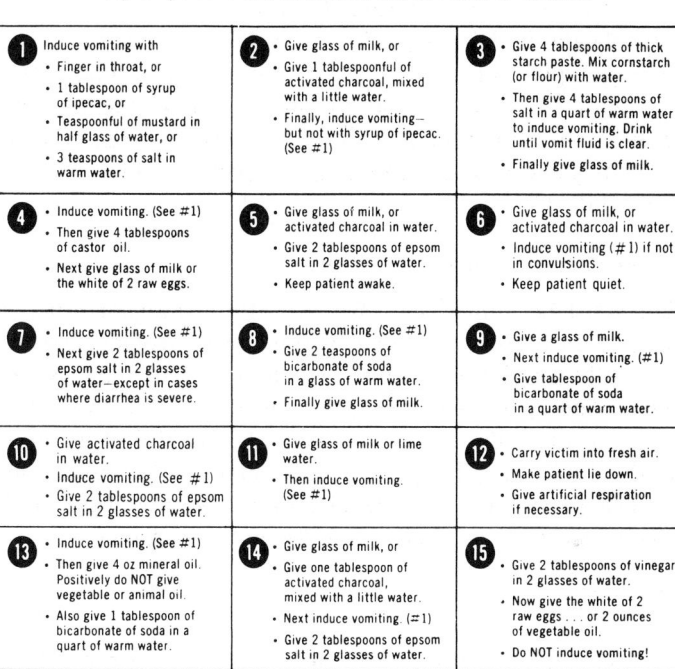

POISONS

- Acids · 18
- Bichloride of Mercury · 14
- Camphor · 1
- Carbon Monoxide · 12
- Chlorine Bleach · 17
- Detergents · 17
- Disinfectant
  - with chlorine · 17
  - with carbolic acid · 4
- Food Poisoning · 7
- Furniture Polish · 16
- Gasoline, Kerosene · 16
- Household Ammonia · 15
- Insect & Rat Poisons
  - with arsenic · 2
  - with sodium fluoride · 11
  - with phosphorus · 13
  - with DDT · 7
  - with strychnine · 6
- Iodine Tincture · 3
- Lye · 15
- Mushrooms · 7
- Oil of Wintergreen · 9
- Pine Oil · 16
- Rubbing Alcohol · 9
- Turpentine · 16

1
- Induce vomiting with
  - Finger in throat, or
  - 1 tablespoon of syrup of ipecac, or
  - Teaspoonful of mustard in half glass of water, or
  - 3 teaspoons of salt in warm water.

2
- Give glass of milk, or
- Give 1 tablespoonful of activated charcoal, mixed with a little water.
- Finally, induce vomiting—but not with syrup of ipecac. (See #1)

3
- Give 4 tablespoons of thick starch paste. Mix cornstarch (or flour) with water.
- Then give 4 tablespoons of salt in a quart of warm water to induce vomiting. Drink until vomit fluid is clear.
- Finally give glass of milk.

4
- Induce vomiting. (See #1)
- Then give 4 tablespoons of castor oil.
- Next give glass of milk or the white of 2 raw eggs.

5
- Give glass of milk, or activated charcoal in water.
- Give 2 tablespoons of epsom salt in 2 glasses of water.
- Keep patient awake.

6
- Give glass of milk, or activated charcoal in water.
- Induce vomiting (#1) if not in convulsions.
- Keep patient quiet.

7
- Induce vomiting. (See #1)
- Next give 2 tablespoons of epsom salt in 2 glasses of water—except in cases where diarrhea is severe.

8
- Induce vomiting. (See #1)
- Give 2 teaspoons of bicarbonate of soda in a glass of warm water.
- Finally give glass of milk.

9
- Give a glass of milk.
- Next induce vomiting. (#1)
- Give tablespoon of bicarbonate of soda in a quart of warm water.

OVERDOSES

- Alcohol · 9
- Aspirin · 9
- Barbiturates · 10
- Belladonna · 6
- Bromides · 7
- Codeine · 5
- Headache & Cold Compounds · 9
- Iron Compounds · 8
- Morphine, Opium · 5
- Paregoric · 5
- 'Pep' Medicines · 2
- Sleeping Medicines · 10
- Tranquilizers · 10

10
- Give activated charcoal in water.
- Induce vomiting. (See #1)
- Give 2 tablespoons of epsom salt in 2 glasses of water.

11
- Give glass of milk or lime water.
- Then induce vomiting. (See #1)

12
- Carry victim into fresh air.
- Make patient lie down.
- Give artificial respiration if necessary.

13
- Induce vomiting. (See #1)
- Then give 4 oz mineral oil. Positively do NOT give vegetable or animal oil.
- Also give 1 tablespoon of bicarbonate of soda in a quart of warm water.

14
- Give glass of milk, or
- Give one tablespoon of activated charcoal, mixed with a little water.
- Next induce vomiting. (#1)
- Give 2 tablespoons of epsom salt in 2 glasses of water.

15
- Give 2 tablespoons of vinegar in 2 glasses of water.
- Now give the white of 2 raw eggs ... or 2 ounces of vegetable oil.
- Do NOT induce vomiting!

16
- Give water or milk.
- Then give 4 tablespoons of vegetable oil.
- Do NOT induce vomiting!

17
- Give patient one or two glasses of milk.

18
- Give large quantity of water.
- Give 2 tablespoons of milk of magnesia.
- Do NOT induce vomiting!

Copyright 1970. *American Druggist* Magazine. Reprinted with permission.

tively small amounts of carbon monoxide in the body will affect certain brain functions, particularly reaction time. The effect that carbon monoxide has upon the individual depends in part on the concentration present, ventilation or fresh air movements, the age, weight, and physical condition of the individual. Some individuals seem quite susceptible to carbon monoxide while others are not as easily affected. Care must be taken during the rescue procedure so that the rescuers themselves are not overcome by the gas. Symptoms generally appear when the blood is 25 percent saturated with carbon monoxide, unconsciousness occurs at 40 to 50 percent, and death at 65 percent.

Indicators of Carbon Monoxide Poisoning

An individual suffering from carbon monoxide poisoning will often be quite unaware that he is being poisoned. He may become dizzy and complain of a headache, find he is unable to walk, feel nauseous, may even be vomiting, complain of a ringing in the ears, a pounding of the heart (due to increased circulation and transport of available oxygen), and feel generally weak muscularly. A lethargy develops, the mucous linings and skin turn a cherry red, and a stupor develops which leads to a coma and eventual death.

First Aid Procedures for Carbon Monoxide Poisoning

The individual must be immediately removed from the contaminated atmosphere and given supportive oxygen therapy. If no oxygen is available, mouth-to-mouth ventilation should be administered until oxygen becomes available. The individual should be given care for shock and transported to a medical facility as soon as possible. Careful observation is necessary as the heart may be permanently affected by the carbon monoxide. However, as in the case with electricity, the first aider must be careful not to be overcome himself while attempting a rescue.

Chlorine Poisoning

Chlorine, an irritant gas when inhaled, causes acute respiratory irritation which may be followed by pneumonia, pulmonary edema, and circulatory collapse. Unlike carbon monoxide, chlorine has a peculiar odor that is easily recognizable. The gas is greenish-yellow, non-flammable, and is widely used in substantial quantities for water purification. Chlorine leaks frequently occur in and around home and public swimming pools.

The indicators of chlorine poisoning are nausea, coughing or gasping for breath, and irritated and painful mucous membranes.

First Aid Procedures for Chlorine Poisoning

Again, as in carbon monoxide instances, care must be taken by the first aider to avoid inhaling the fumes during the rescue effort. Oxygen should be administered, and the affected parts of the body washed with water while the individual is being transported to a medical facility.

Tear Gas

Although tear gas is being included among the inhaled poisons, one might consider it an irritant rather than a poisonous gas, as compared to carbon monoxide. Tear gas and similar lacrimators are chemical mixtures which cause an exposed individual to break out in tears. A warm prickly sensation about the face and neck is also present, and in some cases headache, nausea, and vomiting occur. There is usually no permanent damage and the effects wear off quickly. Because it is highly irritating yet low in toxicity, tear gas is widely favored for riot control use.

If at all possible, remove the affected individual from the contaminated area. If an individual must remain in an area where tear gas is being used, a protective mask should be worn. If irritation persists when the individual has been removed from the contaminated area, cleansing with clear water, especially flowing water over the eyes, seems to be most beneficial.

INJECTED POISONS

Poisonous products may also enter the body directly through injection in the bloodstream. The most common are snake bites, insect bites, and the bites of rabid animals. These injuries and their care are described in Chapter 4. The injection of drugs such as opium, morphine, and heroin in overdoses is discussed in Chapter 10.

ABSORBED POISONS

Some individuals are affected adversely when they are in direct or indirect contact with certain plants. Most common of these irritating plants are poison ivy, poison oak, and poison sumac, poison ivy being the leading culprit. These plants contain a chemical substance which, upon contact with the skin, causes an itching rash to appear. Some individuals are highly susceptible to plant poisoning, while others seem to be naturally immune. But there is no lifetime immunity, and one's resist-

Figure 8.4   POISONOUS CONTACT PLANTS IN THE UNITED STATES

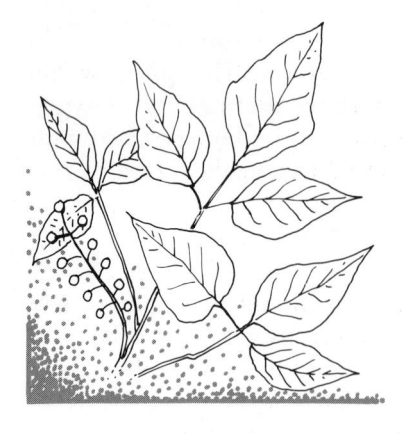

COMMON POISON IVY

- Grows as a small plant, a vine, and a shrub.
- Grows everywhere in the United States except California and parts of adjacent states. Eastern oak leaf poison ivy is one of its varieties.
- Leaves always consist of three glossy leaflets.
- Also known as three-leaf ivy, poison creeper, climbing sumac, poison oak, markweed, picry, and mercury.

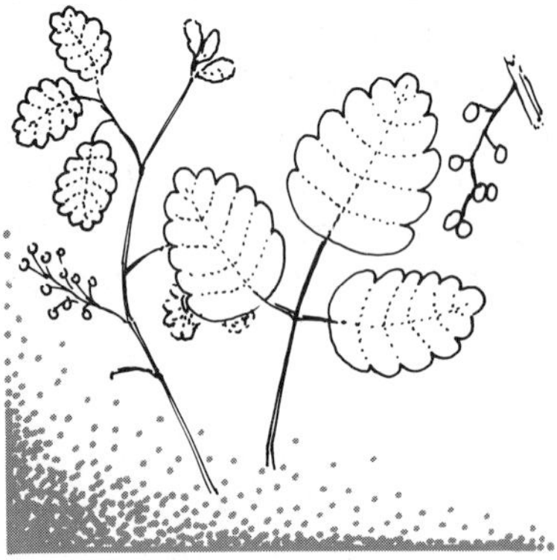

WESTERN POISON OAK

Grows in shrub and sometimes vine form.
- Grows in California and parts of adjacent states.
- Sometimes called poison ivy, or yeara.
- Leaves always consist of three leaflets.

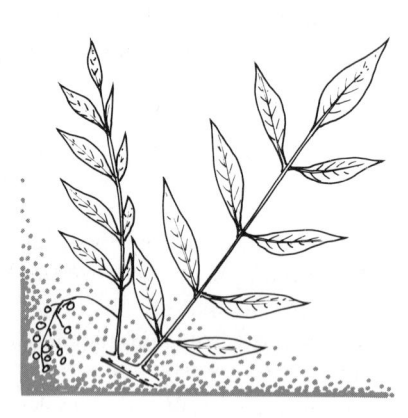

POISON SUMAC

- Grows as a woody shrub or small tree from 5 to 25 feet tall.
- Grows in most of eastern third of United States.
- Also known as swamp sumac, poison elder, poison ash, poison dogwood, and thunderwood.

ance decreases with each exposure. Identification of the plants is important if one is to avoid contact (see Figure 8.4).

Contact Plant Poisoning

If one does come into contact with the plants there is usually a reddening of the skin, with blisters forming which are extremely itchy. If the blisters are broken, it is believed that the fluid will cause the rash to spread. In severe cases, large areas become affected, swelling occurs, and the individual should seek medical attention.

First Aid Procedures for Plant Poisoning

Following contact with toxic plants, one should wash thoroughly with soap and water to remove as much of the irritating substance as possible. Do not open the blisters but use itch-reducing products, which also aid in drying up the blisters. If severe, seek medical attention, as antihistamines and various corticosteroids may be administered under medical supervision.

Lead Poisoning

There appears to be quite an increase in incidences of lead poisoning, particularly among young children. Acute lead poisoning may occur from accidental ingestion of lead salts, but fortunately this is rare. However, chronic lead poisoning—a slow buildup within the body until it finally reaches a toxic level—is increasing to the point of being a leading cause of childhood poison incidents. In the past, lead was used as the base for most paints and may have been used in the water-carrying pipes within homes. Children, particularly young ones, like to chew or suck on the sides of an old crib or toy, window sills, trim, or furniture. Even though these objects may have been repeatedly painted with new harmless water-base paints, the older lead pigments remain and the child absorbs the leaded paint. In addition, old flaking paint, plaster, or wallpaper seem to attract children.

Indicators of Lead Poisoning

Signs of chronic lead poisoning are rather difficult to pinpoint as they reassemble other childhood ailments. The earliest signs include vomiting, constipation, a grayish appearance of the face, in addition to irritability and loss of appetite. The victim may complain of a sweet, metallic taste or dryness of the mouth, and thirst. In severe cases the lead may affect the central nervous system and convulsions may occur in the child. Lead poisoning may cause irreversible damage to the brain, liver, and kidneys.

First Aid Procedures for Lead Poisoning

Even in the mildest case the child should be hospitalized. Treatment is available but requires close medical supervision.

Miscellaneous Absorptions

Many insecticides and pesticides may be inhaled and absorbed into the body with improper use. Usually the affected individual may suddenly lapse into bizarre behavior, collapse, or become unconscious. The first aider should search for any containers, and get the affected individual to medical attention immediately. It may take some time and thorough diagnostic tests to determine what has poisoned the individual.

9

MEDICAL EMERGENCIES

The first aider is often called upon to assist an individual who has not been injured physically or emotionally, but rather is suffering from an acute or chronic illness. In most cases the first aider can do little to assist this individual, except perhaps to recognize the nature of his illness and obtain the medical assistance required. Some of the medically-orientated emergencies frequently encountered are heart attacks, strokes, diabetic reactions, convulsions, epilepsy, acute appendicitis, and unknown unconsciousness. In addition, the first aider may come upon various infectious diseases. These do not usually present a life-threatening situation but must be recognized and receive the proper medical treatment. A chart of the common communicable diseases is included for reference purposes (see Figure 9.1).

GENERAL UNCONSCIOUSNESS

Probably the most frustrating experience a first aider may face is finding an individual in an unconscious state. Unconsciousness is generally described as an interruption of the action of the brain or an unawareness of one's own existence or surrounding environment. Medically, unconsciousness may be differentiated as (a) the comatose state and (b) the stuporous state. Stupor usually indicates partial consciousness, with the mind and senses dulled, whereas coma usually indicates a complete loss

Figure 9.1 COMMON COMMUNICABLE DISEASES

Disease and Cause	Mode of Transmission	Incubation Period	Recognition
Chickenpox *Varicella* virus	Direct contact; droplet spray from sneeze or cough	13 to 21 days	Mild fever; lassitude; skin rash (like blisters)
Diphtheria *Corynebacterium diphtheriae* bacillus	Direct contact; droplet spray from sneeze or cough; skin lesions; carriers; contaminated milk	2 to 5 days	Sore throat; pain; fever; croup; hoarseness; nasal discharge; patches of grayish membrane in nose, throat, and on tonsils
Encephalitis Virus	Mosquitoes; occasionally ticks	5 to 15 days	Sudden onset with high fever; generalized rigidity; headache; muscle pain; upset stomach; respiratory distress; coma and delirium
German Measles *Rubella* virus	Droplet spray from sneeze or cough; contaminated articles	14 to 21 days	Sore throat; headache; fever; tender lumps behind ears; a transient rash
Infectious Hepatitis Unknown agent	Intimate person-to-person contact, fecal-oral contact; transfusion of whole blood; contaminated syringes	15 to 50 days	Fever; nausea; abdominal discomfort followed by jaundice
Influenza Type A, B, and C virus	Direct contact; droplet spray from cough or sneeze	1 to 3 days	Abrupt onset of fever; chills; headache; sore throat; respiratory distress
Measles *Rubeola* virus	Direct contact; droplet spray from mouth or sneeze	7 to 14 days	Fever; rough, red and inflamed eyes; rash starting on face and spreading over entire body
Meningitis Coccus or virus	Direct contact; droplet spray; carriers	2 to 6 weeks	Runny nose; pain in neck and back; sudden onset of fever; loss of alertness; intense headache; nausea and vomiting; may progress to delirium and rash

Figure 9.1 (continued)

Disease and Cause	Mode of Transmission	Incubation Period	Recognition
Mononucleosis Unknown, probably a virus	Unknown; presumably direct contact	Unknown, may be 4 to 14 days	Vague symptoms such as headache, fatigue, sore throat; swollen glands
Mumps Virus	Secretions of the mouth; direct contact; contaminated articles	2 to 4 weeks	Swelling in front of ear; pain on opening mouth; may involve one side or progress to both
Poliomyelitis Virus	Direct contact with infected individual; droplet spray; carriers	7 to 21 days	Irritability; nausea; vomiting; stiffness of neck; muscular soreness; weakness; paralysis
Scarlet Fever Group A hemolytic streptococcus	Droplet infection; direct contact	1 to 5 days	Sore throat; fever; nausea; vomiting; rash
Smallpox *Variola* virus	Droplet spray from cough; body discharge; exude from lesions	7 to 16 days	Sudden onset, fever, chills, headache; backache; rash beginning on face, arms, and wrist; scabs or pocks form later
Strep Throat Group A hemolytic streptococcus	Direct contact; carriers; contaminated dust, food, and articles; secretions from nose and mouth	2 to 5 days	Sudden fever, sore throat; swollen neck glands (same as scarlet fever except for rash)
Tuberculosis *Mycobacterium tuberculosis* bacillus	Droplet infection from nose and mouth; carriers	4 to 6 weeks	Lung lesions diagnosed by X-ray; cough, fatigue; weight loss, hoarseness; chest pain
Typhoid Fever *Salmonella* bacillus	Carriers; infected water; in feces and urine; direct and indirect contact; flies may also spread	1 to 3 weeks	Fever, rose spots, enlarged spleen; diarrhea; headache; constipation; backache; bronchitis; delirium; stupor
Whooping Cough *Bordetella pertussis* bacillus	Droplet spray from cough or sneeze; direct contact	7 to 21 days	Fits of coughing by whoop and vomiting; some fever

Figure 9.2 CLASSIFICATION OF UNCONSCIOUSNESS BY GENERAL APPEARANCE

Condition	Face	Skin	Pulse	Breathing	Eyes	Other Signs
Red Unconsciousness						
Carbon Monoxide	Cherry red	Normal	Rapid and pounding	May have ceased	Normal	
Cerebral Vascular Accident (Stroke)	Red or flushed	Normal, later cool and moist	Slow and strong	Labored—like snoring	Pupils may be unequally dilated	Paralysis; twitching; convulsion
Diabetic Coma	Red or flushed	Dry	Rapid and weak	Air hunger, may be gasping	Normal	Acetone odor on breath. Check for medical ID tag
Heat Stroke	Red	Hot and dry	Rapid and strong	Labored	Pupils may be dilated	High body temperature
Intoxication	Often red; pale to normal	Normal to cool and moist	Strong	Deep or shallow	Pupils normal; eyes red	Odor of alcohol
White Unconsciousness						
Convulsion (Epilepsy)	Pale, some cyanosis	Pale		Sounds labored		Overall muscular twitching; possible loss of bladder and bowel control
Fainting	Pale	Cold and perspiring	Rapid and weak	Shallow	Normal to dilated	Weakness
Frostbite/Exposure	White to grayish yellow	Cold	Normal to rapid	Normal	Normal	Environment:—freezing cold, snow, ice, submersion, wind-chill factor

Heart Attack	Pale to cyanotic	Normal to cool	Weak, rapid to slow	Air hunger, may be coughing or gasping	Normal	Normal to dilated	Pain in chest or left arm
Heat Exhaustion	Pale	Cool and perspiring	Rapid and weak	Shallow	Normal	Normal	Nausea; vomiting, weakness
Hemorrhage (external and internal)	Pale	Cool and perspiring	Rapid and weak	Shallow	Normal to dilated	Normal to dilated	Bleeding from wound or body openings
Insulin Shock	Pale	Moist and cool	Normal	Shallow	Normal to dilated	Normal to dilated	Diabetic? Check for medical ID tag
Poisoning	Pale	Burns or stains on mouth, lips, or hands	Varies	Varies	Varies	Varies	Stomach pain; poison container
Shock	Pale	Moist and cool	Rapid and weak	Shallow	Normal to dilated	Normal to dilated	Restlessness; thirst; trauma evidence
Skull Fracture (Concussion)	Pale	Normal to cool and moist	Strong and slow to rapid and weak	Deep or shallow	Unequally dilated	Unequally dilated	Fluid or blood from facial openings, evidence of blow
Blue Unconsciousness							
Asphyxia—by suffocation	Pale to cyanotic about lips and fingernails	Cool and moist	Weak to absent	Shallow to absent	Normal to dilated	Normal to dilated	
Cardiac Arrest	Pale to cyanotic about lips and fingernails	Cool and moist	Absent	Absent	Dilated and fixed	Dilated and fixed	
Electric Shock	Pale to cyanotic about lips and fingernails	Cool and moist	Rapid and weak to absent	Shallow to absent	Normal to dilated	Normal to dilated	Exit and entrance burns; evidence of power source (electrical cable, rail, lightning)

Medical Emergencies

of response to all external stimuli. The most common causes of unconsciousness—stupor or coma—include shock, poisoning, chemical or drug reactions, head injury, CVA (cerebral vascular accident, also known as stroke or apoplexy), diabetes, fainting, heart attack, or convulsions.

Indicators of Unconsciousness

Upon discovering an apparently unconscious individual, the first aider should immediately check for a medical identification bracelet or medallion. This may indicate the nature of the illness and facilitate prompt treatment. However, if no medical identification is found, the first aider may attempt to determine the level of unconsciousness of the individual. This can be done by (1) attempting to talk to the individual, (2) attempting to draw back the eyelids (an individual in a stupor objects to this procedure, while one in a coma will not react), and (3) observing the response of pupils of the eye (in a stupor the pupils will react to light and constrict, while in a coma the pupils will remain dilated).

The first aider should immediately check to see whether the individual is breathing and his heart is beating or whether these vital functions have ceased. If breathing has stopped and there is no pulse, initiate cardiopulmonary resuscitation procedures as discussed in Chapter 3. If the individual is breathing on his own, observe him carefully and maintain an open airway. Once this has been established, the first aider may look for signs or symptoms which may indicate the nature of the illness, such as the skin color, whether flushed, pale, or bluish-gray (cyanotic). Figure 9.2 describes and classifies various states of unconsciousness according to redness, whiteness, and blueness of the skin. Skin temperature and reaction to pain are also signs that the first aider can ascertain which will help in determining what is wrong with the unconscious individual.

First Aid Procedures for Unconsciousness

Although the first aider can play only a limited role in assisting the unconscious individual, these basic steps are important:

1. Maintain an open airway and begin cardiopulmonary resuscitation if indicated.
2. Position the individual on his side with the head slightly lowered, in case of vomiting. If spinal or head injuries are present or suspected, the individual should not be moved.
3. Check and give care for shock.
4. Administer nothing by mouth if semi-conscious or unconscious.
5. Transport to a medical facility as soon as possible.

DIABETES

Diabetes mellitus, more often referred to as diabetes or sugar diabetes, is a condition in which carbohydrate metabolism is affected due to a deficiency in insulin production or utilization. Insulin is produced in the islets of Langerhans within the pancreas. The true mechanism of insulin action at the cell level is as yet unknown, but researchers believe that it acts upon cell membranes to allow glucose (sugar) to enter and nourish the cell. An individual who has diabetes either does not produce enough insulin or produces more insulin than the body can use. If insulin is insufficient or lacking, blood sugar rises as the cells are not able to use the sugar available to them, thus starving. If there is an overabundance of insulin, blood sugar decreases as the cells use too much sugar and deplete the supply going to the brain. Levels of blood sugar can be analyzed through blood or urine analysis. More women than men seem to develop diabetes. The disease is more common in middle-aged adults, but may occur in young children. Overweight individuals are found to develop diabetes more often than individuals at normal weights. Heredity also is an important predetermining factor. Although there is no known cure for diabetes at present, it is controllable through diet and by taking insulin either by injection or by mouth. Every diabetic should wear a medical identification bracelet or medallion indicating this condition to assure proper treatment in case of emergency. This is very important because diabetics may undergo insulin reactions which if untreated may lead to coma and death. Two conditions may develop—diabetic coma (hyperglycemia) or insulin shock (hyperinsulinism). The comparison chart (Figure 9.3) will help the first aider to differentiate between the two.

Diabetic Coma (Hyperglycemia)

Diabetic coma develops when there is insufficient insulin within the body to allow the cells to utilize the needed sugar. Therefore, blood sugar levels rise and a condition known as acidosis develops. This usually occurs when the individual has eaten excessively or forgotten to take his daily dose of insulin. As the condition progresses the individual becomes confused, disoriented, and may lapse into a coma.

In addition to acting confused and disoriented, the individual may appear as though he has a fever. The skin is flushed and dry, the lips are cherry red in color. Breathing may be spasmodic, and there will be a sweet, fruity odor to his breath. This characteristic odor is acetone (likened to nail polish remover). Due to their flushed appearance and disori-

Figure 9.3 COMPARISON OF DIABETIC REACTIONS

	Insulin Shock (Hyperinsulinism)	Diabetic Coma (Hyperglycemia)
History	Rapid onset following insulin injection	Increasing thirst; air hunger; sleepiness; nausea and/or vomiting
Previous diet	Insufficient food	Excessive food
Insulin	Excessive	Insufficient
Onset	Sudden	Gradual
General appearance	Looks pale and weak	Looks ill or toxic
Fever	Seldom present	Frequently present
Breath	No odor	Acetone (fruity) odor
Skin	Pale and moist	Dry and flushed
Thirst	Absent	Intense
Mouth	Drooling	Dry
Nausea	Seldom	Often
Abdominal pain	Absent	Common
Respiration	Normal	Spasmatic; deep and rapid
Pulse	Normal	Weak and rapid
Blood pressure	Normal to low	Low
Mental state	Possible delirium or deep coma	Gradual development of coma
Trembling	Frequent	Absent
Convulsions	In late stages	None
Treatment	Carbohydrate ingestion	Insulin injection by physician
Response to treatment	Rapid	Slow

Source: William T. Brennan and Donald J. Ludwig, *Guide to Problems and Practices in First Aid and Civil Defense*, 2nd ed. William C. Brown Company, Dubuque, Iowa, 1970.

ented manner, diabetics suffering from hyperglycemia are often accused of being intoxicated. For this reason it is most important for diabetics to wear medical identification to ensure receiving prompt medical treatment.

First Aid Procedures for Diabetic Coma

The individual in a diabetic coma must have insulin if he is to survive. Since an injection of insulin is a medcal procedure, there is little the first aider may do except to transport the individual to a medical facility as quickly as possible. During transport the individual should receive care for shock, and an open airway maintained.

Insulin Shock (Hyperinsulinism)

Insulin shock develops in an individual who has an oversupply of insulin within the body, which allows the cells to use too much sugar and deprives the brain of its due supply. In this condition the level of blood sugar decreases, as opposed to rising in diabetic coma. Hyperinsulinism develops suddenly, usually following a recent ingestion or injection of insulin.

The individual suffering from insulin shock looks much like he is in traumatic shock. The skin is pale and moist and covered with a cold sweat. Respiration is near normal to slow and shallow, while the pulse will be weak and rapid. There is no characteristic odor on the breath as in diabetic coma.

First Aid Procedures for Insulin Shock

Unlike diabetic coma, the first aider may assist the individual suffering from insulin shock, and observe a rapid reversal of symptoms. The individual requires sugar to balance the abundance of insulin present in his body. If conscious, the individual may be given anything containing sugar that the body can absorb quickly. Granular sugar or orange juice are the most rapidly absorbed. If unconscious, place a small amount of sugar or a teaspoon of orange juice on the tongue; consciousness will be regained quickly and then additional sugar may be given. Even though the individual appears to recover, it is recommended that medical attention be sought, as metabolic changes may be occurring within the body requiring an adjustment in insulin dosage.

CONVULSIONS

Convulsions are involuntary muscular contractions or twitchings which may be localized or generalized and may affect one or both sides of the body. Convulsive movements are outward signs of an underlying disease or condition within the body. They may be caused by a CVA (stroke or apoplexy), head injury, communicable disease (particularly in children), abnormal chemical changes in the body, or birth injuries; they may follow periods of anoxia or result from a high fever (particularly in children). Regardless of the underlying cause, the first aider should protect the individual from hurting himself, and seek medical attention as quickly as possible, especially if it is an initial episode. (Further first aid procedures are described below.)

Epilepsy

Epilepsy is probably the most common cause of convulsions. Medically, the term *epilepsy* is applied to a group of diseases characterized by repeated episodes of sudden overactivity of the nervous system. This sudden overactivity manifests itself through uncontrollable involuntary muscular contractions. Approximately one percent of our population, including all age groups, suffers from epilepsy.

Within the brain there are billions of nerve cells which manufacture a supply of electrical energy in order to function. This electrical energy is supplied through chemical action within the nerve cells. Discharge and recharge occur constantly and instantaneously. Medical researchers believe that an epileptic seizure (convulsions) is a sign of abnormal release of energy within the brain. Epilepsy may be caused by a variety of conditions, including childhood infections, birth injuries, concussions, brain injury, scar tissue, and aftereffects of anoxia. Recent research has made available several anti-convulsant drugs which enable the epileptic to lead a fairly normal life. When seizures do occur, they may vary in length and intensity. Four types of seizures commonly occur: *grand mal*, a violent overall seizure; *petit mal*, a brief, less violent seizure; *focal seizure*, where one area of the body or set of muscles twitch; and *psychomotor seizure*, which affects the mental process as well as the muscles. Only through electroencephalograph (EEG) analysis can a true diagnosis be made. First aiders are generally most concerned with grand mal and petit mal seizures, in which the epileptic may require some assistance.

Indicators of Grand and Petit Mal Seizures

Petit mal seizures are characterized by a partial loss of consciousness accompanied by minor convulsive movements of the extremities. The individual is aware of what is going on about him and the seizure generally lasts only a very short period of time.

Grand mal seizures, on the other hand, are characterized by severe, violent convulsions. An individual suffering from grand mal seizures usually has a premonition, or *aura*, that a seizure is about to occur. He loses consciousness, may fall, and begins overall body convulsions or twitching. There may be severe, convulsive spasms of the face muscles and a foaming saliva drooling from the mouth. In severe instances, the individual may vomit and lose bowel and bladder control. His face is livid and the veins of the neck are usually distended. Breathing is usually loud and labored. Often individuals do not breathe for a period of time and may become cyanotic (turn bluish). They will, however, begin breathing on their own once the spasm is over. Seizures usually last only a few minutes, but in rare instances anti-convulsant drugs may need to be administered in order to control the involuntary muscular contractions. Prior to actually convulsing, some individuals seem to "freeze" (tonic state) in position. This may also affect the respiratory system. Spasms usually follow in a short period of time.

First Aid Procedures for Epilepsy

The most important thing that a first aider may do to assist an individual who is suffering a seizure is to prevent the aspiration of vomitus, saliva, or blood. If the mouth is open, place a padded bite stick between the teeth. If the mouth is clenched shut, do not force it open. The stick helps to prevent the individual from biting his tongue and choking on blood and saliva. Under no circumstances should the first aider use his fingers as a bite stick. Try to observe breathing and maintain an open airway in the best way possible. Remove any furniture or objects from around the individual so that he will not strike these objects and harm himself. *Do not restrain* the individual; he will cease convulsing as the brain energy is expended. Upon relaxation of the seizure, the individual may not be aware that he has had a seizure. Do not question him or appear to be overly sympathetic or cause him embarrassment. Always examine the individual for possible injuries that may have occurred as he collapsed or during the seizure. Generally, epileptics wish to rest and sleep following the seizure and should be allowed to do so. Medical attention should be sought in order to insure proper recovery from the seizure.

HEART ATTACKS

The term *heart attack* is a collective phrase used in describing several types of cardiac disorders. Before these disorders can be discussed it is necessary to understand something of the heart organ itself and the disease which affects it.*

The heart muscle (myocardium), like any other muscle, needs a constant supply of oxygen in order to survive and function. This supply of oxygen is provided through the continuous circulation of oxygenated blood from the left ventrical of the heart to the various organs of the body, including the myocardium itself. The only blood supply to the myocardium is provided through two small arteries known as the coronary arteries. Anything interfering with the blood flow through these arteries can cause damage to the heart muscle or even sudden death. Atherosclerosis is a disease which affects the coronary arteries by narrowing these vessels and thus causing interference with the normal blood flow to the heart muscle. This narrowing of the arteries is a result of the deposit of a fatty substance known as plaque on the inner walls of the artery. An individual is said to be suffering from coronary heart disease (CHD) when the condition of atherosclerosis has become so serious that

*For a diagram of the heart, see Appendix B.

the heart muscle is not provided with an adequate supply of blood. Although the cause of atherosclerosis is not yet established, it is a known fact that the disease appears more often in men than in women, in individuals suffering from diabetes, and in individuals whose families have had a history of heart disease. Although coronary heart disease may exist in varying degrees of severity, this chapter will deal with only the more serious forms: coronary insufficiency, myocardial infarction, and congestive heart failure.

Coronary Insufficiency (Angina)

Coronary insufficiency is a condition where the coronary arteries have narrowed to the extent that the blood supply to the myocardium is inadequate. Generally, if the individual is not exerting himself physically, there is a sufficient blood supply to maintain the heart muscle. But when the individual exerts himself physically, there is insufficient oxygen to the heart muscle and he will suffer a chest pain known as *angina pectoris*.

Indicators of coronary insufficiency are sharp chest pain, usually just under the sternum, but the pain may radiate to the left shoulder and arm and occasionally into the neck and jaw. The individual may describe the pain as a feeling of tight pressure, and it is most often felt after exercise, heavy physical activity, eating, temperature variances, or emotional stress.

First Aid Procedures for Angina

Angina pains usually cease if the individual stops the activity engaged in and rests for a short period of time. Many individuals who are diagnosed as subject to angina attacks take nitroglycerine (a small tablet placed under the tongue for rapid absorption). Nitroglycerine dilates the coronary arteries and thus increases the blood supply to the heart muscle. The nitroglycerine takes effect almost instantaneously, and the individual should find relief within a few minutes. But if the pain continues six to ten minutes after resting and taking nitroglycerine, the attack may be more serious, and an ambulance should be called. Under no circumstances should the individual be allowed any physical exertion —even the slightest— or be subjected to emotional stress or upset.

Myocardial Infarction (MI)

Occasionally a blood clot (thrombus) will develop or a piece of plaque (embolus) will become dislodged in a coronary artery and cause a complete block (embolism) to the circulating blood. When this occurs, the affected area will be starved of blood and oxygen, and the surrounding cells of the myocardium (heart muscle) will be destroyed (Figure 9.4). This event is often referred to as a heart attack or a coronary; in medical terminology it is known as an *acute myocardial infarction* (MI). The immediate action which a first aider takes following an acute MI could make the difference between life or death.

As with angina pectoris, chest pain will usually be the first clue that the individual has suffered an acute MI. Unlike angina pain, however, this pain will be continuous and much more intense. The pain will not necessarily begin during physical exertion nor will it cease after a period of rest. The individual may perspire profusely, feel nauseated, and be extremely weak. His face is usually flushed, vomiting may occur, and he may gasp for breath. In addition, the individual is usually apprehensive as he fears impending death.

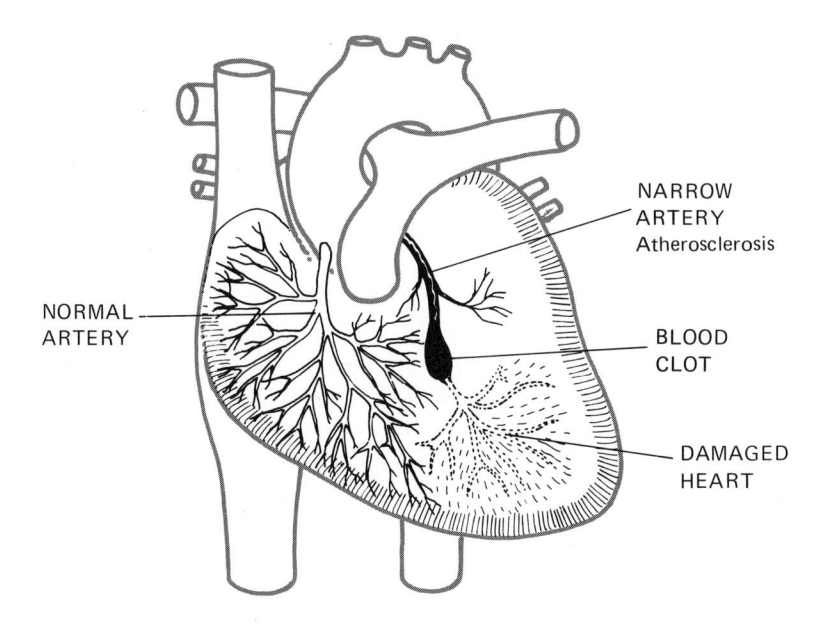

Figure 9.4 Mechanism of a myocardial infarction.

First Aid Procedures for Acute MI

Individuals suspected of suffering an acute MI must be made to lie down and rest at once and must avoid all exertion. They should not be allowed to climb or descend stairs or even to walk to the bathroom. An ambulance should be called immediately to provide proper transportation to a medical facility. If the individual loses consciousness, care as for shock. The first aider must closely monitor the individual's pulse and respiration. Oxygen should be given if available. Should the individual suffer a cardiac arrest, immediate application of cardiopulmonary resuscitation is essential.

Congestive Heart Failure

Congestive heart failure may be caused by a variety of conditions including coronary heart disease, defective heart valves, extreme high blood pressure, or congenital heart defects. The effect is a gradual loss of the heart's pumping effectiveness; however, an "attack" may occur rather suddenly. As the heart's pumping mechanism fails, blood circulation decreases and fluids collect in the tissue surrounding the blood vessels. The resultant condition is called edema (swelling), and most often affects the legs and ankles. In advanced stages of congestive heart failure, pulmonary edema develops. This is a condition where fluids collect in the lungs and cause the individual extreme breathing difficulties. An attack of this type usually occurs suddenly, and the first aider must take positive steps to reassure the individual and make him more comfortable.

The most obvious indication of pulmonary edema will be the individual's extreme breathing difficulty. He will gasp for breath and seek a sitting-up position. His skin will be cyanotic due to inefficient blood oxygenation. Usually there is swelling of the feet and ankles.

First Aid Procedures for Congestive Heart Failure

The primary first aid measure to be initiated is proper positioning of the individual. Because of the large fluid accumulation in the lungs, these individuals will almost always be most comfortable in a semi-reclining position. They should be kept warm and oxygen administered if available. These individuals require immediate medical attention and should be transported promptly by ambulance to a medical facility.

CEREBRAL VASCULAR ACCIDENT (CVA)

Cerebral vascular accident, also known as apoplexy or stroke, occurs when there is a sudden cessation of blood supply to a portion of the brain. Like the heart, the brain needs a constant supply of oxygen in order to survive. An interruption of the blood supply will result in the immediate death of brain tissue. Depending on the vessel affected and the portion of the brain involved, the individual may be left permanently disabled physically and/or mentally. Strokes usually occur as a result of the rupture of an artery in the brain (cerebral hemorrhage), or the occluding of a blood vessel by a blood clot (cerebral thrombosis), or occlusion by foreign matter (cerebral embolism), as shown in Figure 9.5.

Indicators of Cerebral Vascular Accident

The indicators of a CVA will vary depending upon the extent of damage to the brain. If the damage is slight, the individual may only complain of a headache or occasional dizziness. The individual may demonstrate a partial loss of memory or a slight slur in his speech. In the event that extensive brain damage has occurred, the individual may suffer partial or complete paralysis on one or both sides of the body. The pupils of the eye may be unevenly dilated, one side of the mouth may droop slightly, and he may vomit, convulse, lose bladder and bowel control, or become completely unconscious.

First Aid Procedures for CVA

The individual should be made to lie down with his head slightly elevated—never elevate the legs. An ice bag may be placed on the individual's head, but no liquids, and especially no stimulants, should be given by mouth. As with coronary cases, immediate medical attention is necessary. If the individual becomes unconscious, be certain that an adequate airway is maintained.

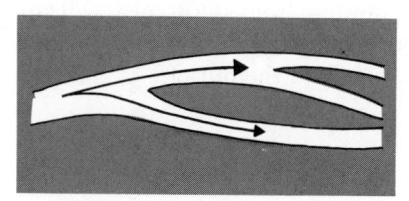

Hemorrhage
The wall of an artery of the brain may break, permitting blood to escape and thus damage the surrounding brain tissue.

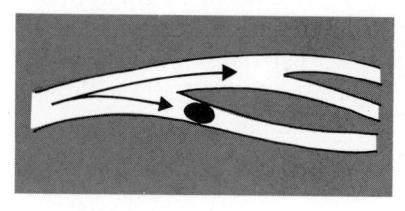

Thrombosis (clot formation)
A clot of blood may form in an artery of the brain and may stop the flow of blood to the part of the brain supplied by the clot plugged artery.

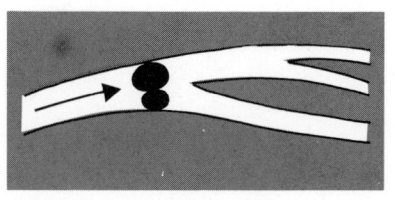

Embolism (blocking of a vessel by a clot floating in the blood stream)
A clot from a diseased heart or, less commonly, from elsewhere in the body may be pumped to the brain and stop up one of the brain's arteries.

Figure 9.5 Mechanism of a cerebral vascular accident.

APPENDICITIS

Protruding from the large intestine is a wormlike projection known as the appendix. The condition whereby the appendix has become inflamed is known as appendicitis. The first aider should always suspect appendicitis when an individual complains of sustained stomach pains, especially with children or adults over age 50.

Indicators of Appendicitis

A typical appendicitis attack begins with pains in the lower abdomen. After two or three hours have passed, the individual will feel nauseated and may vomit. Eventually the pain will become localized in the lower right side of the abdomen. Any attempt to touch this area will cause acute pain. Accompanying high fever indicates a body infection. If these symptoms occur, the first aider should always suspect appendicitis and he should seek medical attention immediately.

The greatest danger from an appendicitis attack is the possibility that the appendix may rupture and cause infection of the abdominal lining, a condition known as peritonitis which, if not treated immediately, will result in death. An individual who is suffering from peritonitis will appear very ill. His skin will be pale and he may appear to be in shock. Pain will have spread to the entire abdomen, and the muscles of this area will be rigid.

First Aid Procedures for Appendicitis

There is little the first aider can do in the handling of appendicitis, but he can take certain steps to make the individual more comfortable. Place the individual in a semi-reclining position with a pillow or folded blanket under his knees. It is most important that the individual not be given food, drink, or laxatives. The use of laxatives, especially with children, could prove to be fatal. Remember that appendicitis can be corrected only through emergency surgery, and no time should be lost in seeking immediate medical attention.

10

PSYCHOLOGICAL EMERGENCIES

Occasionally a first aider may be called upon to assist an individual who is suffering from an alcohol or drug reaction or who has become emotionally disturbed. Recognition of these situations is not always easy since individuals vary considerably in their actions and reactions when exposed to alcohol, drugs, emotional stress, or disaster. However, the first aider must be aware of the possibility of these reactions, care for the indicators present, and seek medical attention for the individual as soon as possible.

EMOTIONAL FIRST AID

There are individuals who suffer a temporary emotional breakdown in reaction to an auto collision, train wreck, plane crash, earthquake, fire, flood, or other disaster. And there are the emotionally disturbed who suffer with a chronic mental illness. Regardless of underlying causes, the observable actions—the outward signs—that disturbed individuals display fall into similar patterns. Some become hysterical, some hallucinate, while others appear withdrawn, quiet, depressed.

Indicators of Emotional Illness

The American Psychiatric Association has classified emotional reactions in disaster and collision situations into five categories: normal, panic, depression, overactive, and physical. Figure 10.1 summarizes the expected reactions of individuals in each of these categories, and gives the techniques which may be employed to assist these individuals. These reactions are for the most part temporary, and with professional assistance the individual returns to a normal state.

Figure 10.1 CLASSIFICATION OF EMOTIONAL REACTIONS

Reaction	Indicators	Assistance Required
Normal	Trembling; muscular tension; perspiration; nausea; mild diarrhea; urinary frequency; pounding heart; rapid breathing; anxiety.	Give reassurance; attempt to motivate; talk with individual; watch for return of composure; do not show resentment or oversympathize.
Panic (flight reaction)	Unreasoning attempt to flee; loss of judgment; uncontrolled crying; hysteria; wild running about.	Show firmness; isolate if necessary; empathize; encourage to talk; don't overstep your limitations (may need professional help); do not use harsh restraints or douse with water.
Depression (underactive reaction)	Standing or sitting without moving, talking, or showing emotions; vacant or dazed expression.	Attempt to contact and obtain rapport. Try to talk out what happened. Be empathetic; recognize feelings of resentment. Perhaps give a small task to perform. Do not oversympathize, pity, or act resentful. Don't tell them to "snap out of it."
Overactive	Argumentative; rapid, often incoherent talking; short attention span; jumps from activity to activity.	Let them talk; may be able to perform small task. Do not argue or suggest they are acting.
Physical (conversion reaction)	Severe nausea and vomiting; may be unable to speak or move some parts of body.	Show interest; find a small task they can perform to take mind off situation; make comfortable. Treat apparent injury or illness, and transport to a medical facility. Do not blame, ridicule, or ignore disability.

Individuals suffering from more serious and chronic emotional disorders may exhibit a variety of indicators depending upon the illness. These indicators include a sudden change of behavior, strange loss of memory, delusions of grandeur, paranoia (thinking someone is plotting against you), hearing voices, and seeing visions. The most seriously ill may lose all contact with reality. Generally these individuals require professional psychiatric assistance and the first aider, in recognizing this, must act accordingly.

First Aid Procedures

The assistance given to the emotionally disturbed must vary with the individual and the particular circumstances. There is no one way to assist emotionally disturbed individuals. It is a one-to-one situation in most instances. There are, however, a few points which the first aider must keep in mind when dealing with emotionally disturbed individuals.

1. *Recognize the possibility of an emotional injury.* Physical injury is easy to recognize, whereas an emotional injury may not be immediately apparent. The first aider should watch for individuals who appear frightened, anxious, hysterical, dazed, or devoid of emotions.
2. *Keep calm.* Excitement on the part of the first aider may only make things worse. Emotions often transfer. If the first aider appears calm and acts as if he knows what is going on, this may transfer to the disturbed individual and as a result help to calm him.
3. *Recognize your limitations.* The first aider must realize he is there only to assist, not to judge or diagnose. If the situation is beyond his control, professional help in the form of ambulance personnel, police, and so on must be called immediately.
4. *Keep in contact.* Attempt to gain a rapport with the disturbed individual. This is best done with a steady flow of conversation. Let the individual understand that you are trying to help him. Talk in a quiet, calm manner and be truthful, not deceptive.
5. *Avoid excitement.* If necessary, remove the individual from the situation. Further excitement or fright may only make things worse.
6. *Listen.* If the disturbed individual wishes to talk, let him do so. This may vent his emotional tension. However, do not take anything he says personally.
7. *Take your time.* Speed is not necessary. Take the time necessary to calm the individual prior to transporting to a medical facility.
8. *Avoid restraints.* The first aider may need to be firm but should not be harsh in handling hostile individuals. This may be accomplished through the voice directing the individual to do something. If this is not successful, mild restraint, enough to prevent the individual from harming himself or others, may be necessary. Formal restraints such as cuffs, ties, etc., should only be used by law-enforcement agents or physicians.
9. *Transport to a medical facility.* Upon arrival, various medications in the form of tranquilizers and sedatives may be administered by a physician.

ALCOHOL REACTIONS

Intoxication

Consumption of beverages containing ethyl alcohol often leads to a state in which the individual becomes intoxicated or poisoned. In an intoxicated state the individual does not react as he would when he is sober and often becomes involved in collision situations or may cause himself or others bodily harm. It is estimated that approximately 50 percent of auto fatalities involve alcohol consumption. The more an individual consumes, the greater the risk of his becoming involved in a collision.

Upon ingestion, alcohol acts primarily on the central nervous system, that is the brain, where its presence can often be detected within a minute of ingestion. The effect upon the brain depends upon the concentration of alcohol present. The most serious consequences of alcohol use are due to the effect alcohol has upon judgment, inhibition, and reaction time. Alcohol is a depressant and its effect is to make the entire body react more slowly. Individuals are considered legally intoxicated in most states when their alcohol blood level reaches 0.10 percent (one-tenth of one percent). In order to reach this level the average individual (approximately 150 pounds) would need to consume approximately five ounces of 80 proof alcohol in one hour's time. However, even smaller amounts of alcohol present in the body will adversely affect it. Consumption of 2½ ounces of 80 proof alcohol in one hour will bring the alcohol blood level to 0.05 percent—at which level body impairment is evident in most individuals. There are several variables which determine the blood level of alcohol in an individual. They include body weight, strength (proof) of the alcohol, stomach contents (type and amount of food present), and rate of alcohol consumption. Several alcohol blood level charts are available for determining the amount of liquor one needs to consume to reach various alcohol blood levels. Figure 10.2 provides data for both an empty and full stomach.

Indicators of Intoxication

The most prominent indicator of an intoxicated individual is the odor of alcohol on the breath. The individual may be conscious or partially or totally unconscious. In the early stages of intoxication, the individual's face appears flushed and moist, his pulse is strong and his breathing deep. As the concentration of alcohol in the blood rises, his face becomes dry and bloated, and the pulse becomes weak, while breathing becomes shallow. The eyes appear bloodshot and equally dilated. If conscious, the individual may stagger and his speech will be slurred.

Psychological Emergencies   [155]

Figure 10.2   APPROXIMATE AMOUNT OF 80 PROOF LIQUOR NEEDED TO REACH GIVEN LEVELS OF ALCOHOL IN THE BLOOD

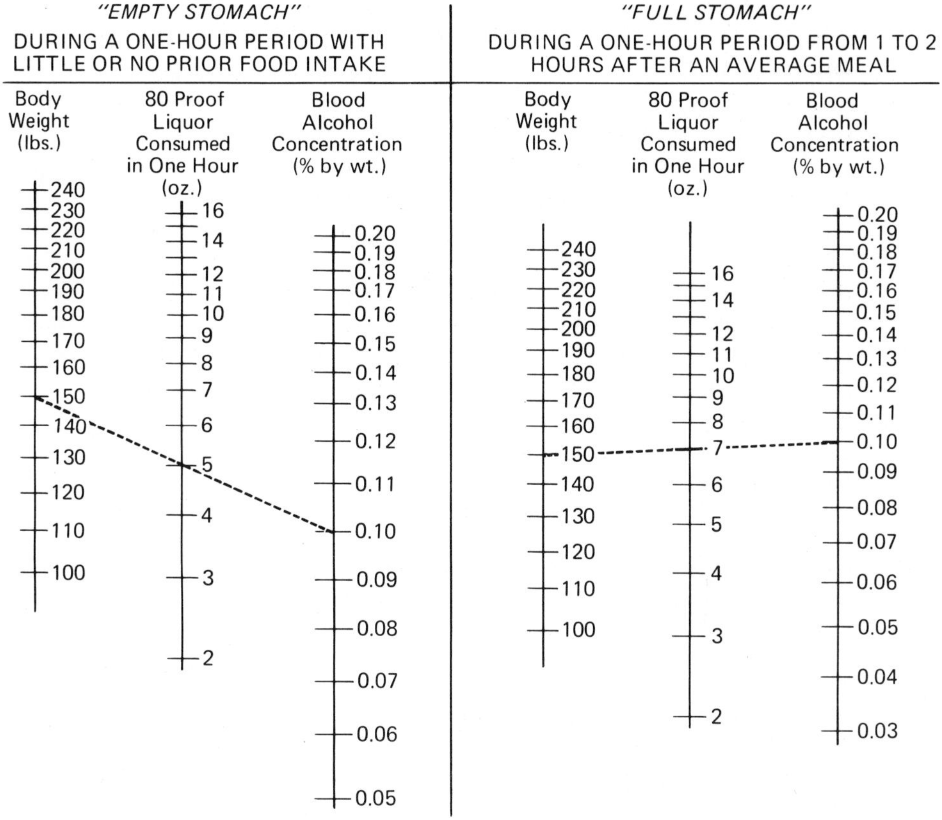

"EMPTY STOMACH"
DURING A ONE-HOUR PERIOD WITH LITTLE OR NO PRIOR FOOD INTAKE

Body Weight (lbs.)	80 Proof Liquor Consumed in One Hour (oz.)	Blood Alcohol Concentration (% by wt.)
240	16	0.20
230	14	0.19
220	12	0.18
210	11	0.17
200	10	0.16
190	9	0.15
180	8	0.14
170	7	0.13
160	6	0.12
150	5	0.11
140	4	0.10
130	3	0.09
120	2	0.08
110		0.07
100		0.06
		0.05

"FULL STOMACH"
DURING A ONE-HOUR PERIOD FROM 1 TO 2 HOURS AFTER AN AVERAGE MEAL

Body Weight (lbs.)	80 Proof Liquor Consumed in One Hour (oz.)	Blood Alcohol Concentration (% by wt.)
240	16	0.20
230	14	0.19
220	12	0.18
210	11	0.17
200	10	0.16
190	9	0.15
180	8	0.14
170	7	0.13
160	6	0.12
150	5	0.11
140	4	0.10
130	3	0.09
120	2	0.08
110		0.07
100		0.06
		0.05
		0.04
		0.03

To determine the amount of alcohol to be consumed for one's body weight, locate the body weight and draw a line to the blood level percent desired. For example, on an empty stomach, a 150-pound person would need to consume 5 ounces of 80 proof liquor within one hour to reach a 0.10 percent alcohol blood level. (Adapted from charts prepared by the U.S. Department of Health, Education and Welfare and by the Royal Canadian Mounted Police.)

Psychological Emergencies

First Aid Procedures for Intoxication

As the odor of alcohol may often be confused with that of acetone in a diabetic, the first aider should always check for any medical identification indicating diabetes. The first aider should also check for physical injuries such as hemorrhage and fractures, particularly if the individual has fallen and appears unconscious. If these conditions are found, the proper care for such injuries should be given and the individual transported to a medical facility.

If the individual is simply intoxicated, sleep is probably the most beneficial treatment. Care should be taken, however, not to place the individual on his back. If vomiting occurs, as it often does, the vomitus may be aspirated into the trachea and respiration may be obstructed. Therefore, the individual should be placed on his side with the head slightly lower than the body, as previously discussed for the care of unconscious individuals. If the individual is unconscious and appears seriously intoxicated, he should be transported to a medical facility immediately.

If the individual is conscious and it is desirable to sober him up, there are a few points to keep in mind:

1. The body metabolizes alcohol at a rate of one ounce per hour. This cannot be altered, no matter what is done.
2. If the individual has not already vomited, cause him to do so. This will rid the body of the alcohol remaining within the stomach and reduce the amount to be metabolized.
3. Following vomiting, black coffee with sugar may be administered. This should not be depended upon, however, to sober the individual. This can only be done as the body metabolizes the alcohol present in the blood stream.
4. Handle as for shock, keeping the individual warm and comfortable.

Delirium Tremens

If an individual is an extremely heavy drinker and ceases to consume alcohol for one reason or another, he may develop a disorder known as delirium tremens or D.T.'s. The first signs include a shaking or tremor of the hands, restlessness, and possible auditory and visual hallucinations. The condition may progress to a point of total confusion and disorientation.

First Aid Procedures for D.T.'s

There is really very little the first aider may do to assist an individual who is suffering from D.T.'s except to make him comfortable and transport him to a medical facility.

DRUG REACTIONS

Drug abuse has become a major problem in recent years. Cases of drug overdoses are a common occurrence among young people. Yet drugs in themselves, when taken under medical supervision, need not necessarily be dangerous. When used indiscriminately or in large doses on a regular or increasingly greater basis, then drug abuse exists.

Drugs may be classified into eight groups: alcohol, sedatives, tranquilizers, narcotics, stimulants, cannabis, hallucinogens, and miscellaneous. Figure 10.3 summarizes the various types of drugs, with their characteristics and effects, and gives the specific indicators of drug reactions. The services of the first aider, however, may not be called upon until the drug abuser has overdosed and is in distress. In this case the individual may be in a semi-conscious or unconscious state, suffering from respiratory distress, or may already have stopped breathing.

First Aid Procedures for Drug Abuse

It is the first aider's responsibility to do everything possible to assist the drug abuser without making any value judgment of the circumstances surrounding the incident. As with poisoning, the first aider should care for the indicators that he observes. If the drug has been ingested and the individual is conscious, then the first aider may induce vomiting. If the individual is unconscious, the first aider must maintain an open airway, as discussed in Chapter 2. In severe cases of drug overdose, the affected individual may have suffered a cardiopulmonary arrest. In these instances resuscitative measures must be initiated.

The first aider may encounter an abuser who is hallucinating. In this instance he should handle the individual as he would the emotionally disturbed.

SUICIDE

It is estimated that over 20,000 persons commit suicide annually in the United States. Estimates of unreported statistics, however, place the figure closer to 100,000. Suicide is the fifth leading cause of death in the 15 to 24 age range, and during recent years the suicide rate for young men and women has showed a marked increase. The tragedy lies in the fact that these are all unnecessary and preventable deaths. It is not the intent of this chapter to explain the psychology of suicide, but some of the more common characteristics generally found in potential suicides will be mentioned in order to make the first aider more aware of this problem.

Figure 10.3 IDENTIFICATION OF ALCOHOL AND DRUG ABUSE

Type and Name	Slang Names	Method of Taking	Effects and Dangers	Spotting Abusers
Alcohol	Booz, hooch, juice, sauce, hardstuff	Swallowing liquid	Depressant to central nervous system. Causes relaxation, drowsiness; impaired judgment, reaction time, coordination; frequently aggressive behavior.	Odor on breath; loss of equilibrium and general drunken behavior. Nausea and vomiting in some.
Sedatives Barbiturates	Downers, barbs, blue devils, yellow jackets, dolls, red devils, phennies, goofers	Swallowing pills or capsules	Sluggishness; faulty judgment. Physically addictive. Danger of death in overdose, especially in combination with alcohol.	Thick, slurred speech; appearance of drunkenness with no odor of alcohol. Sedation with variable incoordination.
Tranquilizers	Quieters, downers	Swallowing pills or capsules	Drowsiness, nausea. Possible physical dependence from excessive doses.	Generally same as barbiturates.
Narcotics Heroin Opium Morphine Codeine Demerol Methadone Cough Syrup	Op, horse, H, smack, junk, skag	Smoking (inhalation); injecting in muscle or vein	Euphoria, then drowsiness. Likelihood of physical addiction. Painful withdrawal.	Watery eyes, constricted pupils; calm, inattentive, "on-the-nod" with slow pulse and respiration. Needle marks on arms or body.

Stimulants Amphetamines Methamphetamines Cocaine Preludin	Uppers, pep pills, bennies, cartwheels, crystal, speed, meth, dexies, coke, snow.	Swallowing pills or capsules; injecting in veins; sniffing or injecting.	Abnormal alertness and aggressiveness; loss of appetite. Paranoid activities; acute depression as dose wears off ("crashing"); rapid tolerance build-up. Hyperactivity; possible convulsions	Rapid speech, giggling, loud laughter, an almost abnormal cheerfulness; hyperactive; jumpiness and irritability.
Cannabis Marijuana Hashish	Pot, grass, tea, weed, stuff, hash, joint, reefer, maryjane.	Smoking (inhalation); swallowing.	Euphoria; increased pulse rate. Some alteration of time perception, possible impairment of judgment and coordination. May bring on impulsive behavior, anxiety, or acute panic reactions.	May feel exhilarated or relaxed, stare off into space, be hilarious without apparent cause, have exaggerated sense of ability; dilation of pupils, red eyes. Sweet odor present where smoking.
Hallucinogens LSD Psilocybin STP DMT Mescaline (Peyote)	Acid, sugar, mushrooms, cactus, sunshine, peyote, mesc.	Swallowing liquid, capsule, pill or sugar cube. Smoking, chewing plant.	Hallucinations; unusual hilarity; intense anxiety; impairment of normal motivation can produce panic reaction. Occasional reoccurrance. Swings in mood from high to low.	Behavior may be irrational. Visual imagery, increased sensory awareness, nausea. Impaired coordination.
Miscellaneous Glue Gasoline Solvents		Inhalation.	Produces high with impaired coordination and judgment. May produce some serious liver or kidney damage.	Slurred speech and dulled senses; vision and hearing may be impaired. Bag for inhalation may be found.

Source: *Principles of First Aid: Instructor's Guide*, Robert J. Brady Company, Bowie, Md., 1973.
Note: The effect of any drug depends, among other things, on its strength, the amount taken, and the manner and frequency of use.

Indicators of Potential Suicide

Often an individual exhibits certain signs which should alert those around him that he may attempt suicide. These signs usually are characterized by depression and the various emotional states associated with depression such as disappointment, disillusionment, loneliness, pessimism, and despair. He may talk of committing suicide. If he does he must be taken seriously. This could be a disguised cry for help and it should not be treated lightly or dismissed. The potential suicide may suddenly show a lack of interest in areas that he was greatly interested in or in areas where he formerly performed well. An example is a good student who suddenly does poorly. There may be dramatic changes in communications patterns and an inability to talk about his depression. He may lose contact with his friends and become withdrawn. He may change his daily living patterns, for example, find it hard to fall asleep at night or to wake up and get going in the morning. The potential suicide may also show a change in his social behavior, including the serious use of alcohol or drugs, promiscuity, and temper outbursts.

Of course, a person demonstrating some of these characteristics is not necessarily a potential suicide, but the more characteristics present, the higher the risk that he may attempt suicide. Often a potential suicide will suddenly show an abrupt improvement. This period, it is believed, could be the most dangerous as he may have decided that he has found the solution to his problems by committing suicide.

First Aid Procedures for Potential Suicides

Potential suicides are in need of psychiatric assistance. If the first aider finds himself in a situation where an individual demonstrates suicidal characteristics, it is important that he try to put the individual in contact with someone with whom he can honestly discuss his feelings—a close friend, family member, school counselor, or clergyman. Most colleges and universities and many cities and counties throughout the United States now operate 24-hour suicide prevention or crisis centers. The individual could be placed in contact with one of these centers if immediate assistance is needed. The first aider must recognize his limitations and realize that, as with injuries, he can only assist until professional help can be obtained.

Indicators of Attempted Suicide

Suicide is attempted by a variety of methods, the most common of which are overdoses of barbiturates or sedatives, carbon monoxide or natural gas, shooting, jumping from high places, and hanging. Occasionally the suicide victim will leave a note giving more positive indication that it is a suicide. Regardless of the method of attempted suicide, the first aider will have to administer life-sustaining first aid until an ambulance or rescue squad arrives or until the individual is transported to a medical facility.

First Aid Procedures for Attempted Suicides

The first aider must care for the observed indicators. For example, if the individual has lacerated himself, then the first aider should care for hemorrhage as discussed in Chapter 3. Besides performing the obvious first aid procedures, the first aider must not make any value judgments regarding the circumstances associated with the attempted suicide. If the individual is conscious, every effort should be made to reassure him and inspire his confidence. Onlookers and the curious should be kept away. Care must be taken that the individual not cause further injury to himself or to the first aider. Proper legal authorities should always be notified in the case of attempted suicide.

{ 11 }

EMERGENCY CHILDBIRTH

Occasionally the first aider is called upon to assist in the delivery of a baby. Although not an everyday occurrence, it is an unforgettable experience. The procedures to follow are simple—nature herself does most of the work. In over 95 percent of the cases the emergency delivery will be normal. Women who suffer from prolonged or obstructed labor usually have time to get to a medical facility prior to delivery, while those who emergency deliver usually have short, easy, normal deliveries. The information in this chapter is designed to help the first aider, should he be called to assist during the delivery of a baby.

DEVELOPMENT OF THE BABY

A child is ready to be born approximately 280 days or forty weeks after the last normal menstrual period. Premature births are not uncommon in emergency situations, although those under thirty weeks usually do not survive. The baby has been developing within the uterus, or womb, of the mother. Figure 11.1 illustrates the baby's relationship with the reproductive organs during pregnancy. Within the uterus the baby floats in the amnion, or bag of waters. The amnion serves the following functions: (1) it protects the baby from blows; (2) it allows for freedom of movement; (3) it keeps the baby at an even temperature; (4) it helps to enlarge the vaginal canal prior to delivery, and (5) it acts as a lubricant and disinfectant for the vaginal canal prior to delivery. The baby receives

[164]   Emergency Childbirth

oxygen and nourishment and disposes of waste through the umbilical cord and placenta. The placenta is a three-lobed organ approximately 8 inches in diameter and 1 inch thick. The umbilical cord is twisted like a rope and is approximately 2 feet long. If the cord should become pinched or knotted at any time during pregnancy the baby will receive no oxygen and die within a few minutes. The mouth of the uterus is sealed during pregnancy with a thick mucous plug. This becomes very soft and elastic prior to delivery, and during the labor process it opens (dilates) to allow the baby to move into the vaginal canal toward the outside world.

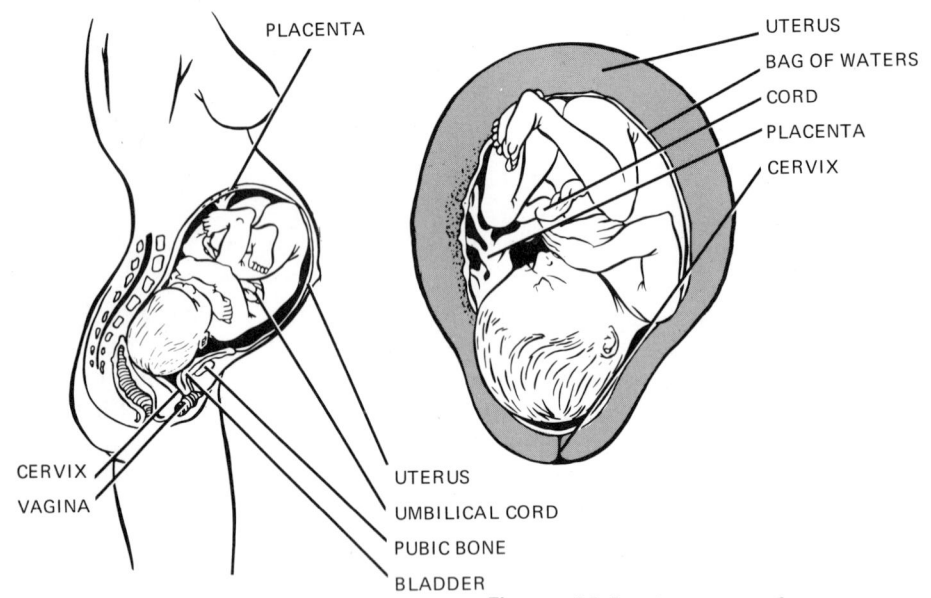

Figure 11.1   Anatomy of pregnancy.

THE BIRTH PROCESS

Birth is a natural process divided into three phases: (1) dilation, (2) expulsion or delivery, and (3) placental expulsion.

Phase One: Dilation

Dilation of the cervix or mouth of the uterus begins the labor process. The onset of labor differs among women, but generally the mucous plug displaces and is seen on the clothing or in the toilet. The length of phase one of labor varies considerably. In first-child deliveries this phase may average 15 to 18 hours, longer in some women. With the second delivery and subsequent births labor is shorter, averaging less than eight hours and sometimes only one and a half hours. Labor pains or contractions, are caused by the rhythmical tightening and relaxation of the muscles of the uterus pulling the cervix open. Contractions progress in frequency, usually occurring at 10-minute, 4-minute, 3-minute, 2-minute, and possibly 1-minute intervals. Each contraction usually lasts 20 to 60 seconds. The strength of the contraction increases as the cervix opens to about four inches, large enough to allow the baby's head to pass through. Figure 11.2 illustrates this opening process. Contractions are involuntary and

(a)

(b)

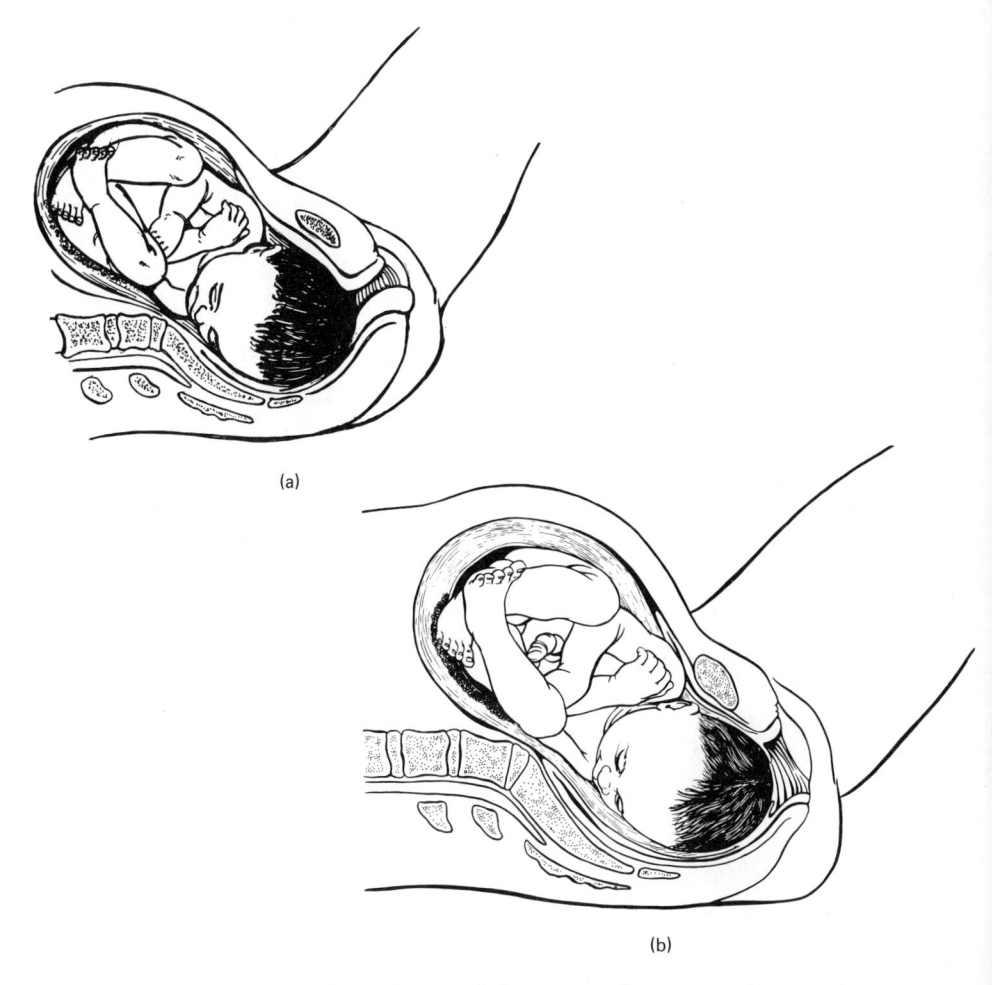

Figure 11.2 During the first phase of labor, muscular contractions open the cervix for delivery. Note the difference in cervix openness (a) early in labor, and (b) at the beginning of delivery.

the mother should not attempt to bear down during the contraction. She should relax as much as possible throughout the first phase of labor. The first aider assists in this phase by making the mother as comfortable as possible and offering words of reassurance. When a first aider comes upon a woman who indicates that she is in labor he should try to determine: (1) how long she has been in labor; (2) the interval between contractions; (3) whether the bag of waters has broken; (4) whether there is bleeding from the vagina; (5) duration of labor in previous pregnancies; and (6) the individual's age (generally, the younger the woman, the easier the delivery).

Phase Two: Expulsion or Delivery

Once the cervix is completely dilated the baby is ready to slide into the vagina, or birth canal. The mother begins to feel as though she were going to have a bowel movement. This sensation comes from the pressure of the baby's head on the rectum. You might explain this to her, but do not let the woman go into the bathroom as she may have the baby in the toilet. Delivery is near when (1) labor pains are strong and one to three minutes apart; (2) the mother attempts to bear down with each contraction; (3) there is a sudden increase in vaginal fluid; and (4) a bulge appears at the vaginal entrance. The bag of waters may break at any time during the first or second phase of delivery, but its rupture generally signals the beginning of the second phase of labor. Approximately one pint to one quart of fluid and blood-stained mucus may be expelled forcefully or may seep out slowly. The vagina is now ready for the baby to slide through. The mother should be lying on her back with knees drawn up (Figure 11.3).

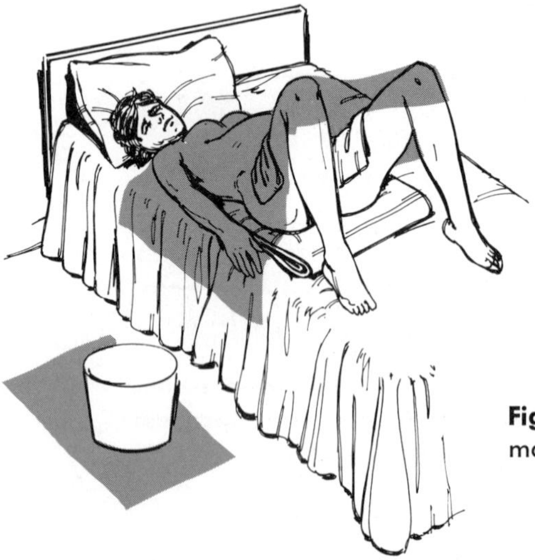

Figure 11.3 Normal position for mother during delivery.

Emergency Childbirth [167]

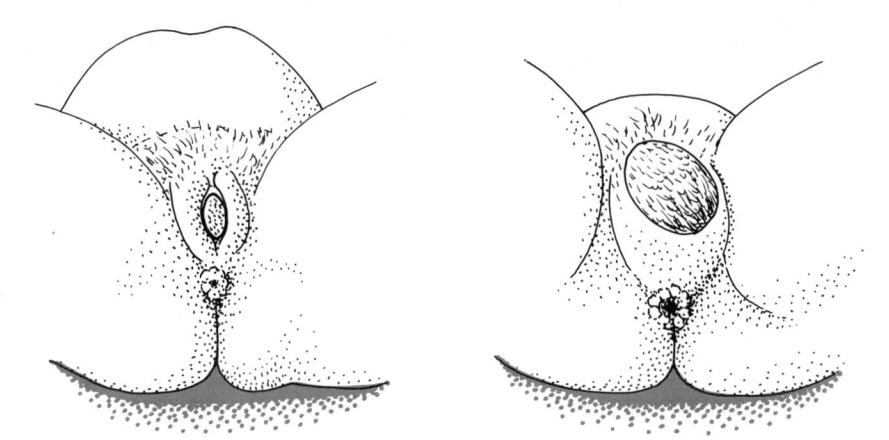

Figure 11.4 During contractions the baby's head will gradually appear. "Crowning" refers to initial appearance of the baby's head.

In a normal delivery, usually the first sign of the baby will be the top of its head which begins to appear with each contraction (Figure 11.4). This is termed *crowning*, and the baby will usually deliver during the next two or three contractions. It is important that the head not pop out too quickly. The assisting first aider may press his fingers against the perineum (the skin portion between the vagina and rectum) and place his hand gently on the infant's head, which will allow the infant to emerge slowly with each contraction. The baby's head is usually born facing downward but quickly rotates so that it faces the mother's thigh, enabling the shoulders to be delivered (Figure 11.5).

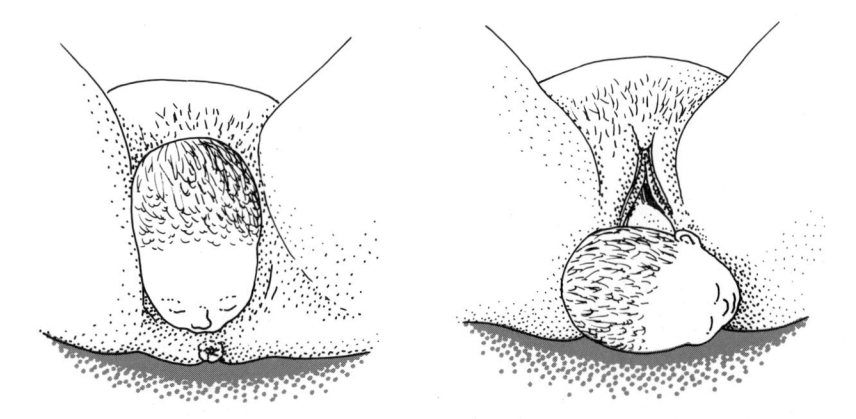

Figure 11.5 As contractions continue, the baby's head will emerge face downward and then rotate to the left or to the right.

(a) (b)

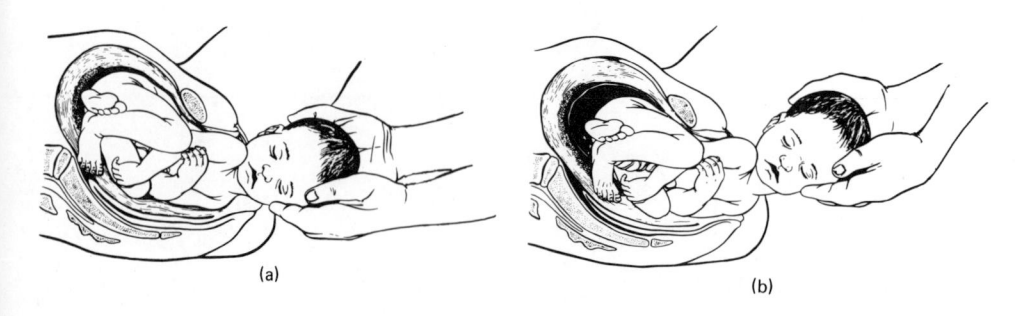

Figure 11.6 If there is difficulty delivering the shoulders, a slight downward movement of the head will assist the upper shoulder to emerge (a), and a slight upward movement of the head will assist the lower shoulder (b).

Approximately one minute following delivery of the head, another contraction will allow the shoulders and rest of the body to deliver. Occasionally the mother may have difficulty delivering the shoulders due to their width. If this is the case, the first aider may assist slightly to ease delivery. As the top shoulder is usually the first to present itself, slight downward pressure on the baby's head (toward the floor) will help deliver the upper shoulder (Figure 11.6a). The back shoulder may be assisted by slight upward pressure on the baby's head (Figure 11.6b). Following the delivery of both shoulders, the rest of the body will deliver effortlessly and quickly. During the entire birth process, the first aider must support the baby on his arms so the baby will not slip. This may be difficult as the baby is covered with a slippery waxy substance which acts as a protection. As soon as the head is delivered, the first aider should check the position of the umbilical cord by feeling about the neck for the cord. If it is wrapped around the neck, quickly loosen it or slip it over the baby's head to prevent strangling (Figure 11.7).

Care of the Infant

Once fully delivered the baby will usually appear purplish-blue, exhibit good muscular tension, and resist external efforts to move his arms and legs. Generally the infant will breathe and cry within two or three minutes. The baby should be securely held by the ankles and back. Elevate the baby's body enough to allow drainage of mucus from the chest and throat (Figure 11.8). Wipe the mouth with a piece of gauze if available and pull the tongue forward to open the air passage. If the baby does not begin to breathe within two or three minutes, check the mouth and nasal area for mucus and clean out again.

Do not slap the baby in an attempt to get him to breathe. Instead, the first aider may try stroking the back vigorously, or stroking from the bottom of the neck toward the chin (in the direction of the arrow in

(a) (b)

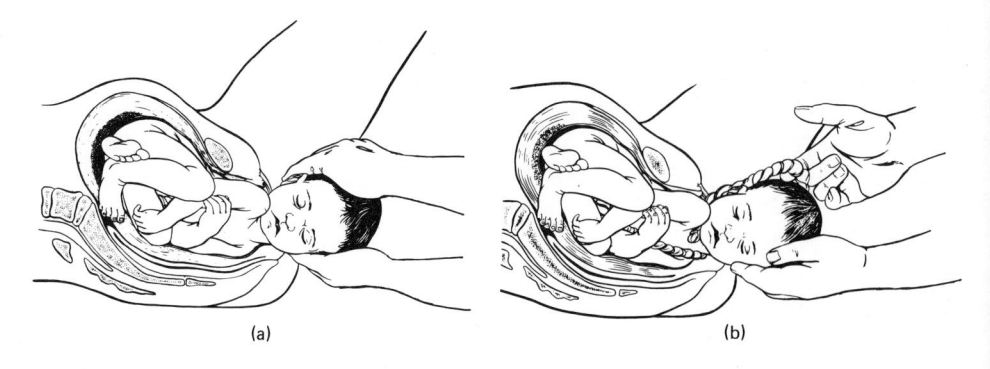

Figure 11.7 As the baby's head emerges it should be gently supported as shown (a) and the position of the cord should be checked immediately (b).

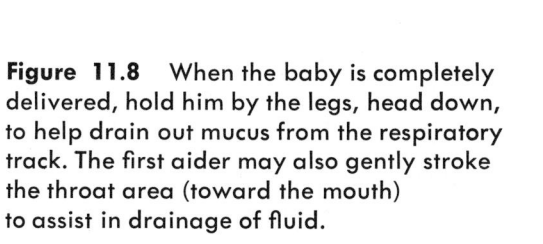

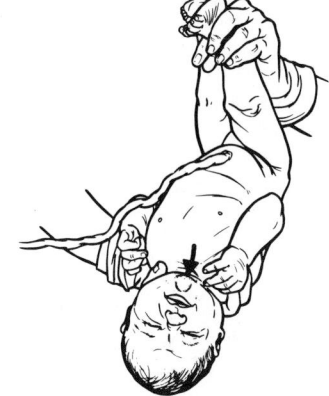

Figure 11.8 When the baby is completely delivered, hold him by the legs, head down, to help drain out mucus from the respiratory track. The first aider may also gently stroke the throat area (toward the mouth) to assist in drainage of fluid.

Figure 11.8), or tapping the soles of the feet in an attempt to get the baby to breathe. If breathing still does not start, begin mouth-to-mouth-and-nose ventilation immediately. Mouth-to-mouth-and-nose ventilation must be done very gently, with short puffs, at a rate of 20 per minute. Usually within a few puffs the child will begin to breathe. In emergency deliveries, babies rarely fail to breathe quickly on their own.

Wrap the baby in a warm blanket and lay him on his side on the mother's abdomen or between her legs. There is no need to cut the umbilical cord until after the placenta has been expelled. There is no reason to do anything to the baby's eyes or to attempt to clean him.

Phase Three: Placental Expulsion

The third phase of labor, expulsion of the placenta, usually occurs a few minutes after delivery of the child (Figure 11.9), although there have been instances of expulsion hours later. Contractions, which cease following the birth of the baby, will return as the uterus begins to expel the placenta. There is no great hurry for this to occur, and under no circum-

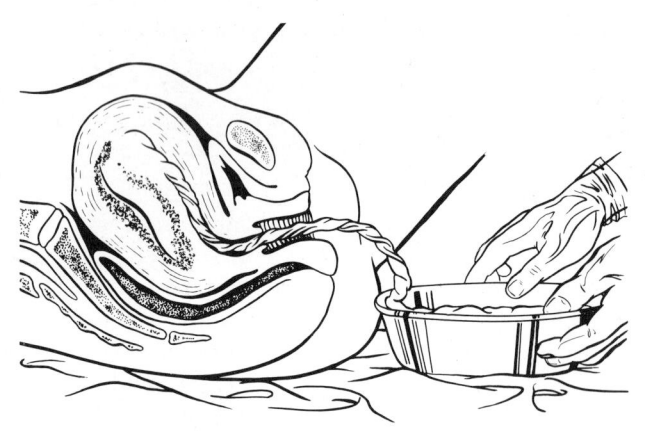

Figure 11.9 Expulsion of the placenta, the third phase of delivery, occurs from several minutes to an hour after the delivery of the baby.

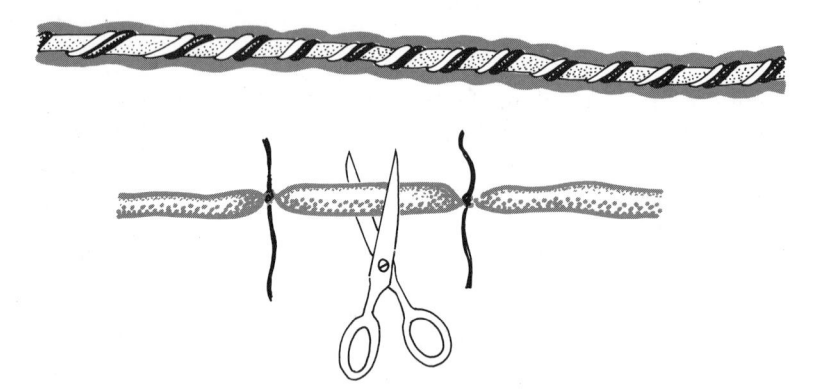

Figure 11.10 After the baby has been delivered and the umbilical cord has ceased pulsating, the cord may be tied off in two places and then cut, as illustrated.

stances should anyone pull on the cord. Once the placenta has peeled itself off the uterine wall and delivered, the mother may bleed, sometimes severely. A sanitary napkin may be used to absorb the discharge, and the uterus may be gently massaged through the abdominal wall by grasping and kneading it gently until it becomes firm. The uterus will feel like a large grapefruit and must contract internally in order to stop hemorrhaging. This may take as long as an hour, and the massaging should continue until the mother arrives at a medical facility.

The placenta must be retained for medical examination in order to determine whether the entire placenta has been expelled. After expulsion of the placenta a decision may be made as to whether to cut the umbilical cord. There is no real necessity to cut the cord immediately, but if it will be some time before the mother and baby reach a medical facility, the cord may be severed.

About five minutes after delivery the umbilical cord will cease to pulsate and may be safely tied and cut. No attempt should be made to cut the cord until this pulsation has ceased. The cord should be tied off in two places with clean flat strips of cloth about the width of shoelaces. One tie is secured approximately four inches from the baby's abdomen and the second is tied two inches further away (Figure 11.10). The knots must be tied securely or the baby may hemorrhage when the cord is cut. The cord is then cut between the two knots, using a scissors, knife, or other sharp, clean instrument. The cord end attached to the baby should be covered with a sterile dressing to prevent infection.

PRE-BIRTH EMERGENCIES

In addition to the problem of hemorrhage which has already been mentioned, other problems may arise during pregnancy or at delivery time. The first aider should be alerted to these difficulties and know what actions he can perform to assist both mother and child.

If an expectant woman develops an illness during her pregnancy, she should be tended for the illness symptoms present, with no undue immediate concern for the unborn child. However, since the woman may be apprehensive for her baby, the first aider can offer comfort and reassurance at this time.

If a pregnant woman is injured in an accident, her injuries should be cared for in accordance with their observable signs. But a serious accident might cause a woman to go into labor prematurely, in which case she should be transported to a hospital immediately. Following any injury, even minor, it is recommended that a pregnant woman see her obstetrician.

DELIVERY COMPLICATIONS

During actual delivery if certain complications arise, there are specific procedures for the first aider to follow.

Arm or Single Leg Presentation

If instead of the baby's head appearing first, a leg or arm is presented (Figure 11.11), the child cannot be delivered without professional assistance. When a hand or arm is presented, this indicates that the baby is lying crosswise within the uterus, with shoulder and arm pointing downward and the head shoved off to one side. When a single leg appears, the baby's body might be positioned correctly for delivery but one leg might be trapped. In either case, the doctor will have to use instruments to turn the baby in order for it to be delivered; or he may have to perform a Cesarean section. Therefore, if you see an arm or leg emerging first rather than the head, cover it with a clean towel and transport the mother to a medical facility as quickly as possible.

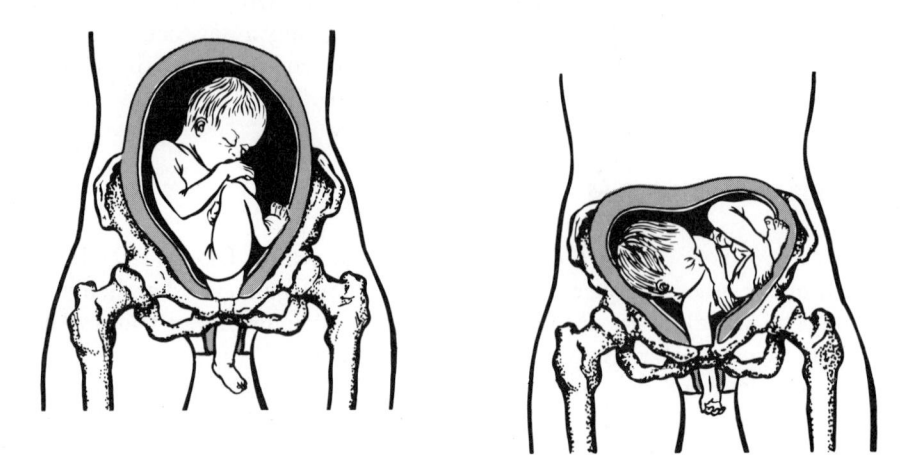

Figure 11.11 In an arm or single leg presentation, no delivery should be attempted. The mother should be transported to a hospital immediately.

Breech Presentation

When both feet (footling) or buttocks (breech) present themselves first in the delivery process, delivery is usually slow and the woman will generally arrive at a hospital before giving birth. Only about four percent of deliveries are breech or footling presentations, and they are not as complicated as is often feared. Since such births are usually premature, the baby is relatively small, which eases the delivery. The major complication in breech and footling deliveries is that the baby's head may compress the umbilical cord during the delivery process and constrict the flow of oxygen to the baby.

The woman should be placed in knee-chest position, on her hands and knees (Figure 11.12), rather than in the normal delivery position (on back with knees drawn up). This reverse position adds the weight of the baby

Emergency Childbirth [173]

to the force of gravity, helping the delivery process. This is not an easy position for the mother to maintain, so she should be assisted throughout the delivery process.

The first indication that it may be a breech delivery is the appearance of the baby's feces, usually dark green, coming from the mother's vagina. The mother usually has little or no difficulty in bearing down with the contractions and pushing the baby out as far as its navel. At this point the first aider may either assist in completion of the delivery or, if in doubt, support the baby and transport the mother to a hospital.

If the baby is small, the mother may have little difficulty in completing the delivery by herself. But if the delivery from the navel to the armpit takes more than two contractions, assistance may be necessary. The first aider who has decided to assist in completion of the delivery should do

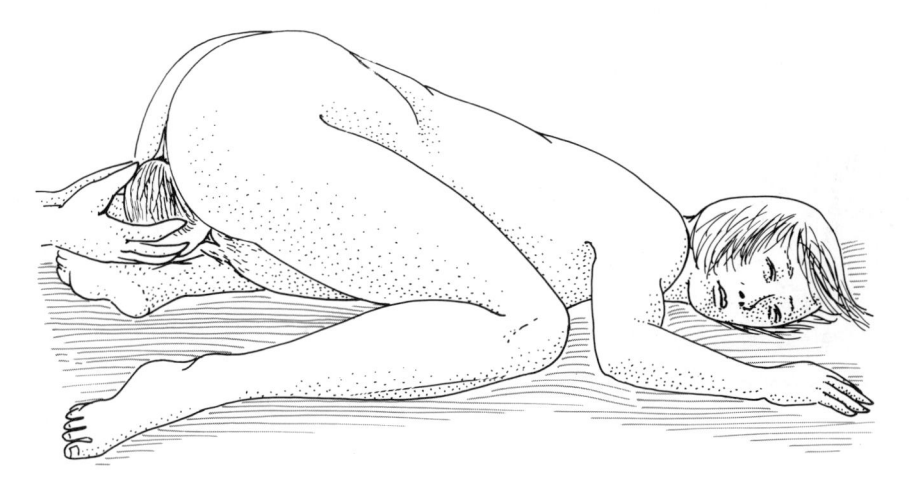

Figure 11.12 Knee-chest position for breech delivery or prolapsed cord.

so very gently and without any haste. The baby's arms should be delivered prior to the head, using either of the following procedures (Figure 11.13): (1) One finger of the first aider can push the shoulder blade toward the baby's spine, which usually causes the arm to drop; or (2) With two fingers the first aider may slide up along the baby's upper arm, grasp the arm and slide it down across the chest and out. Deliver the arm closest to the mother's back first, then the other arm. Once the arms have been delivered, a finger may be inserted in the baby's mouth and the chin can be inclined down toward the chest. This usually permits the head to be delivered.

If the head will not emerge the first aider should open an airway for the baby because it must have oxygen in three or four minutes or anoxia

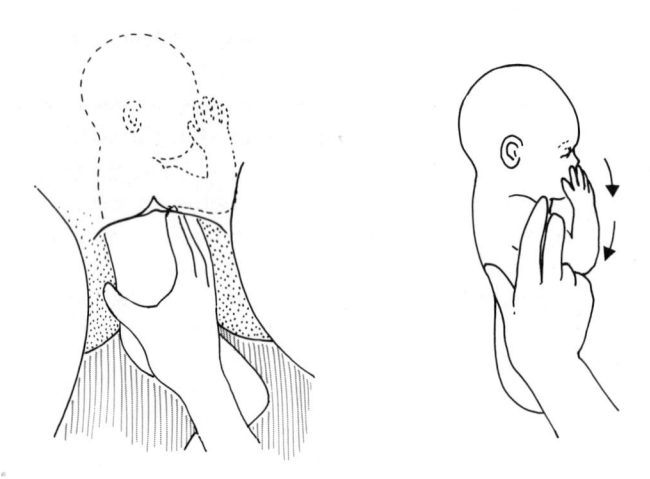

Figure 11.13 Assisting delivery of the arm in a breech presentation.

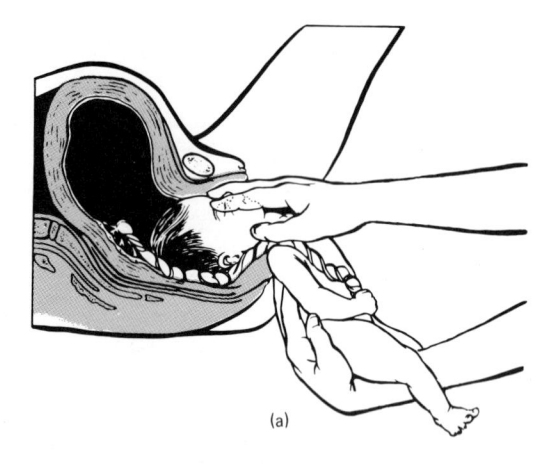

Figure 11.14
Maintenance of an airway in a breech delivery.

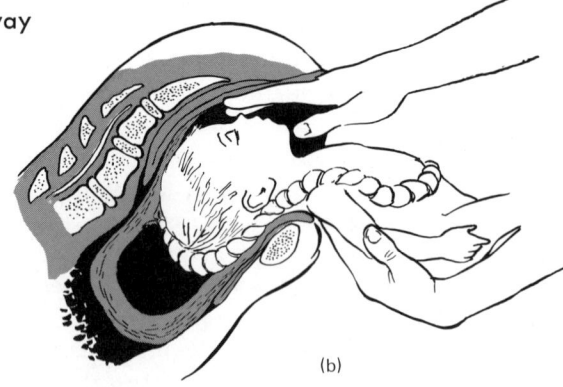

may cause permanent brain damage. An airway may be opened by inserting the index and middle fingers into the vaginal canal. The fingers should be separated around the baby's nose and pushed upward, freeing the baby's face from the vaginal wall (Figure 11.14). This will open an airway and the baby may be supported in this manner until a physician can complete delivery.

Prolapsed Cord

Occasionally, the umbilical cord presents itself prior to the baby's head. As the umbilical cord is the baby's lifeline, compression of the cord during delivery deprives the baby of oxygen and the baby may suffer brain damage or death from anoxia. To prevent compression of the cord the knee-chest position (Figure 11.12) is recommended, although it is difficult for the mother to maintain. This position will allow the weight of the baby to shift off the compressed cord. An alternate method is to place the woman in the position for shock, with the hips and feet elevated 12 to 16 inches. This will cause the baby to drop back into the uterus and remove the pressure from the cord (Figure 11.15). Oxygen should be administered to the mother if available. If still exposed, the cord should be covered gently with a sterile dressing and the mother transported to a medical facility as quickly as possible.

Multiple Births

Each birth in a multiple birth situation should be handled as an individual delivery and the procedures discussed for normal deliveries should

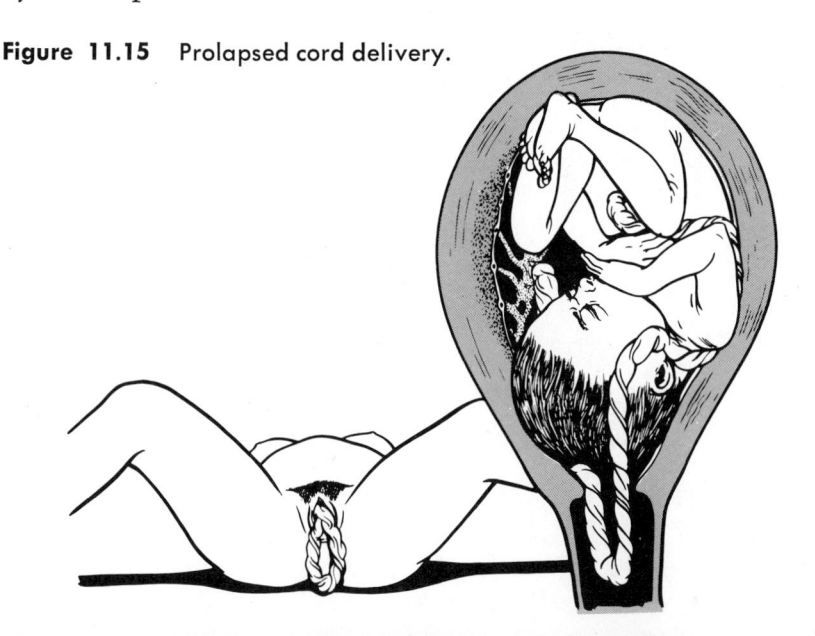

Figure 11.15 Prolapsed cord delivery.

[176] Emergency Childbirth

SEPARATE PLACENTAS

ONE PLACENTA

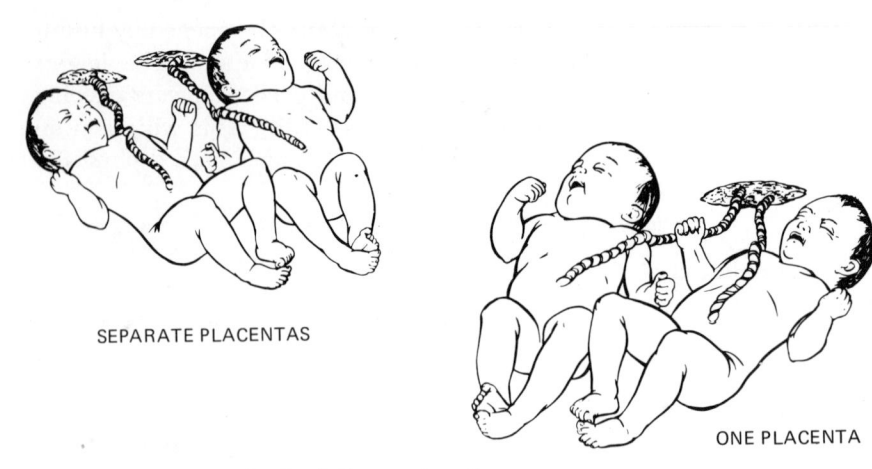

Figure 11.16 Multiple delivery situations.

be followed. After the first baby arrives, each succeeding infant may follow in quick succession or there may be intervals of time before all the deliveries are completed. The infants may share one placenta or have separate placentas (Figure 11.16). Multiple birth babies are often premature and usually small, which facilitates delivery. During the delivery process, the first aider should tie each umbilical cord tightly following delivery so that hemorrhage will not occur with the succeeding babies. It is not necessary to sever the cord—just tie it securely. Second deliveries may be breech, so this should be anticipated and the procedures discussed for breech presentation should be followed.

Abortion (Miscarriage)

Abortion or miscarriage—the expulsion of the fetus prior to its ability to live on its own—may occur at any time from conception to just prior to normal delivery. Usually it occurs during the first three and a half months of pregnancy. The expulsion may be partial or complete and may

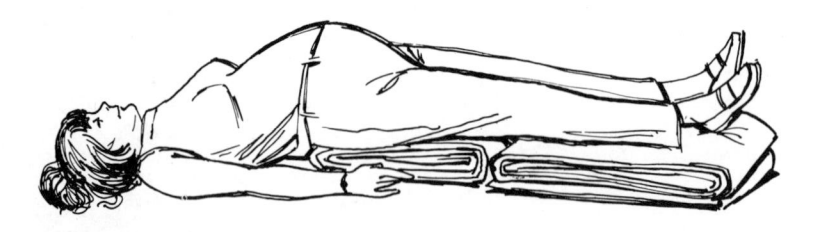

Figure 11.17 Position for hemorrhaging woman in miscarriage.

be accompanied by hemmorrhage and discharge of tissue and blood clots. A woman who is miscarrying (aborting) generally appears to be in shock. Her pulse is fast, she is pale and perspiring, may complain of abdominal cramps, and be too weak to stand. The woman should be kept quiet and placed in shock position with the hips and feet elevated 12 to 16 inches (Figure 11.17). Sanitary napkins may be used to absorb the discharged fluid, which should be retained for medical analysis. Transport the woman to a medical facility as quickly as possible.

{12}

FIRST AID PRACTICAL SKILLS

The practical skills of first aid are vitally important in the care of the injured. This chapter discusses bandaging, splinting, and transport methods that are widely used. These techniques should be practiced regularly by the first aider, so that when needed in an emergency their application becomes almost automatic.

BANDAGING

Bandaging is a relatively easy technique to master. An effective bandage need not be tied as neatly as those illustrated in this chapter; in fact, under emergency situations it may be difficult, if not impossible, to take the time to tie a perfectly neat bandage. What is important in bandaging is that a bandage must not be secured so tightly that it cuts off circulation, yet must be tight enough to control hemorrhage or to stabilize a fracture. Bandaging techniques must be practiced over and over until the first aider is able to apply a bandage correctly without hesitation. By learning a few basic bandaging techniques, the first aider should be able to improvise and bandage just about any part of the body.

The two basic types of bandages are the roller gauze bandage and the triangular bandage (termed a *cravat* when folded). Other common forms of bandaging materials include adhesive strips (Band-Aids), elastic wraps, and adhesive tape (Figure 12.1). When these materials are not

[180]   First Aid Practical Skills

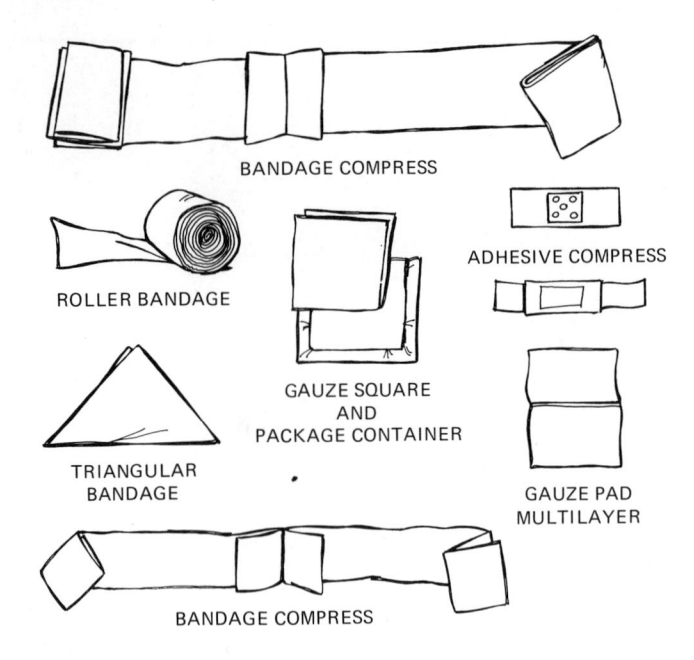

Figure 12.1   Types of bandages.

available, the first aider may improvise by using a clean handkerchief, towel, cloth, a piece of clothing, or even a belt.

Bandages are used primarily for the following purposes:

1. To provide direct pressure over a wound for control of hemorrhage.
2. To prevent contamination of a wound by holding a sterile dressing (compress) in place.
3. To immobilize a fracture by holding splints in place.

Before any type of bandage is applied, certain preparations should be made in the area to be bandaged. The wound or laceration should first be covered with a sterile dressing. These dressings are available in a variety of sizes, the most common ranging from 2-inch to 4-inch squares. Larger pads for covering massive wounds are also available. Sufficient dressings should be applied in relation to the severity of the hemorrhage. If there is no hemorrhage, one or two layers of dressing should be sufficient. If hemorrhage is more severe, then many layers will be necessary in order to increase absorption. Care should be taken when unwrapping dressings from their packaging so that the sterile surface does not come into contact with the first aider's hands and thus become contaminated. Once a dressing comes into contact with the affected area, it should be left in place. It should not be moved into another position as this will spread contamination. If the dressing is off-center, just apply additional dressings rather than move the misplaced one. The dressing should be large enough to extend at least an inch beyond the edges of the wound.

Roller Gauze Bandages

A roller gauze bandage consists of a long strip of gauze material which has been rolled into a cylinder. It can be purchased commercially in a variety of widths and lengths and, as it is often sterile, it can be applied directly to a wound if a sterile compress is not available. A newer type of roller gauze is made of a soft fabric that stretches and is self-adhering. This material is excellent as it conforms to irregular surfaces such as joints, and also facilitates splinting.

The application of a roller gauze consists of three steps: (1) anchoring the bandage, (2) applying the bandage, and (3) securing the bandage.

Anchoring the Bandage

A roller gauze must first be anchored so that it stays firmly in place. If an arm or leg is being bandaged, for example, anchoring is accomplished by starting the end of the bandage at an angle to and above the first layer of roller gauze. After encircling the extremity twice, fold the protruding end down and continue to encircle the extremity (Figure 12.2). Once the bandage is firmly anchored, the next step is to apply successive layers of gauze.

Applying the Bandage

The most common and versatile forms of roller gauze bandages are the *spiral turns*, which can be either complete spirals (also called *circular turns*), closed spirals, or opened spirals.

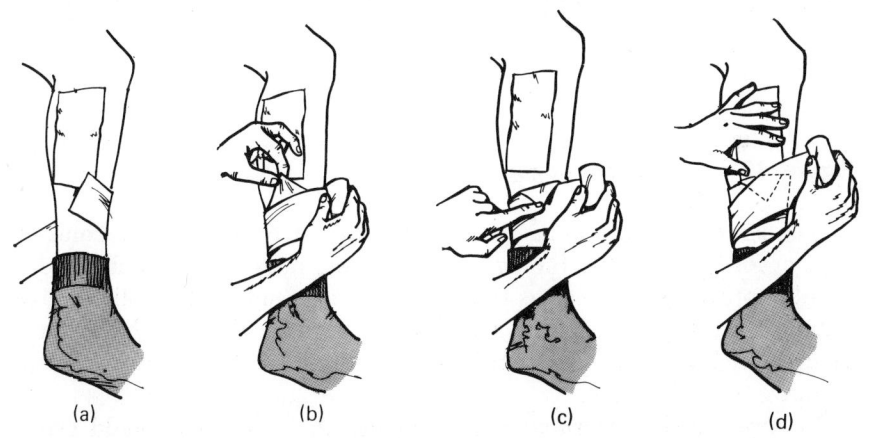

(a) (b) (c) (d)

Figure 12.2   Anchoring the roller gauze.

In a complete spiral each layer of gauze completely overlaps the underlying layer (Figure 12.3a). In a closed spiral each layer of gauze overlaps the underlying layer by one-half its width (Figure 12.3b). And in an open spiral the layers do not overlap but are separated so that the skin or dressing is exposed between the spirals (Figure 12.3c). The open spiral bandage does not apply a great amount of pressure and should be used to secure a dressing covering a large area where hemorrhage is not severe. It is particularly useful for holding large dressings over burned areas.

(a) COMPLETE SPIRAL

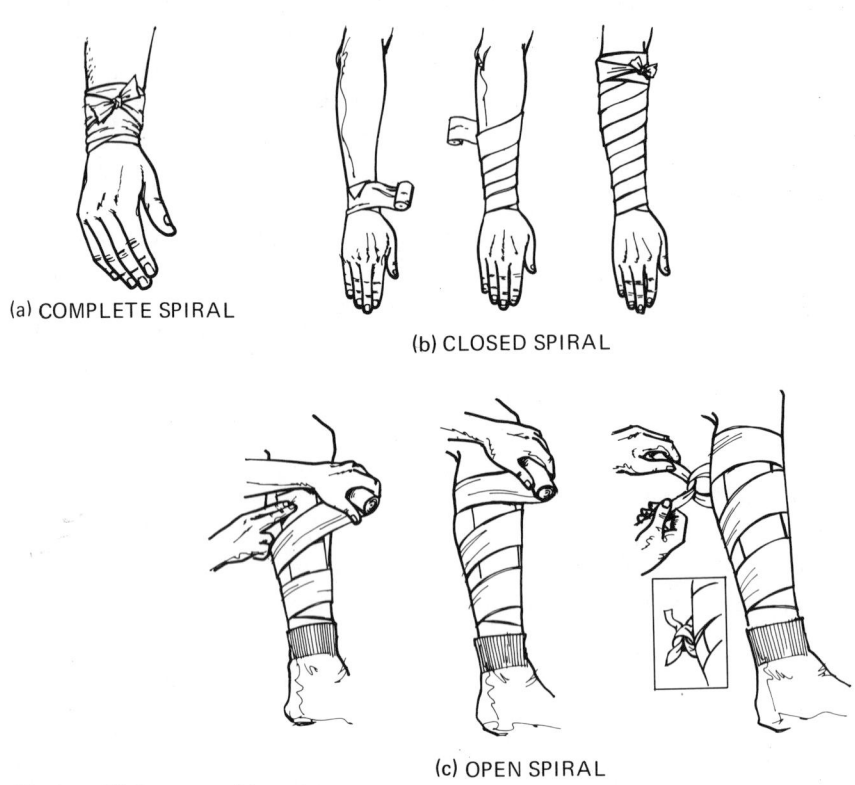

(b) CLOSED SPIRAL

(c) OPEN SPIRAL

Figure 12.3 Spiral bandages.

The *figure-of-eight bandage* is most useful for bandaging the hand or foot, or for joints such as the wrist, ankle, knee, and elbow. The first aider should apply sterile dressings to the wound, then anchor the roller gauze with several complete spirals. Continue by making diagonal layers in a figure-of-eight pattern as illustrated in Figure 12.4. Be careful to make all turns uniformly tight.

In applying the *recurrent finger bandage* the first aider should use a

(a) HAND

(b) KNEE

(c) FOOT

Figure 12.4
Figure-of-eight bandages.

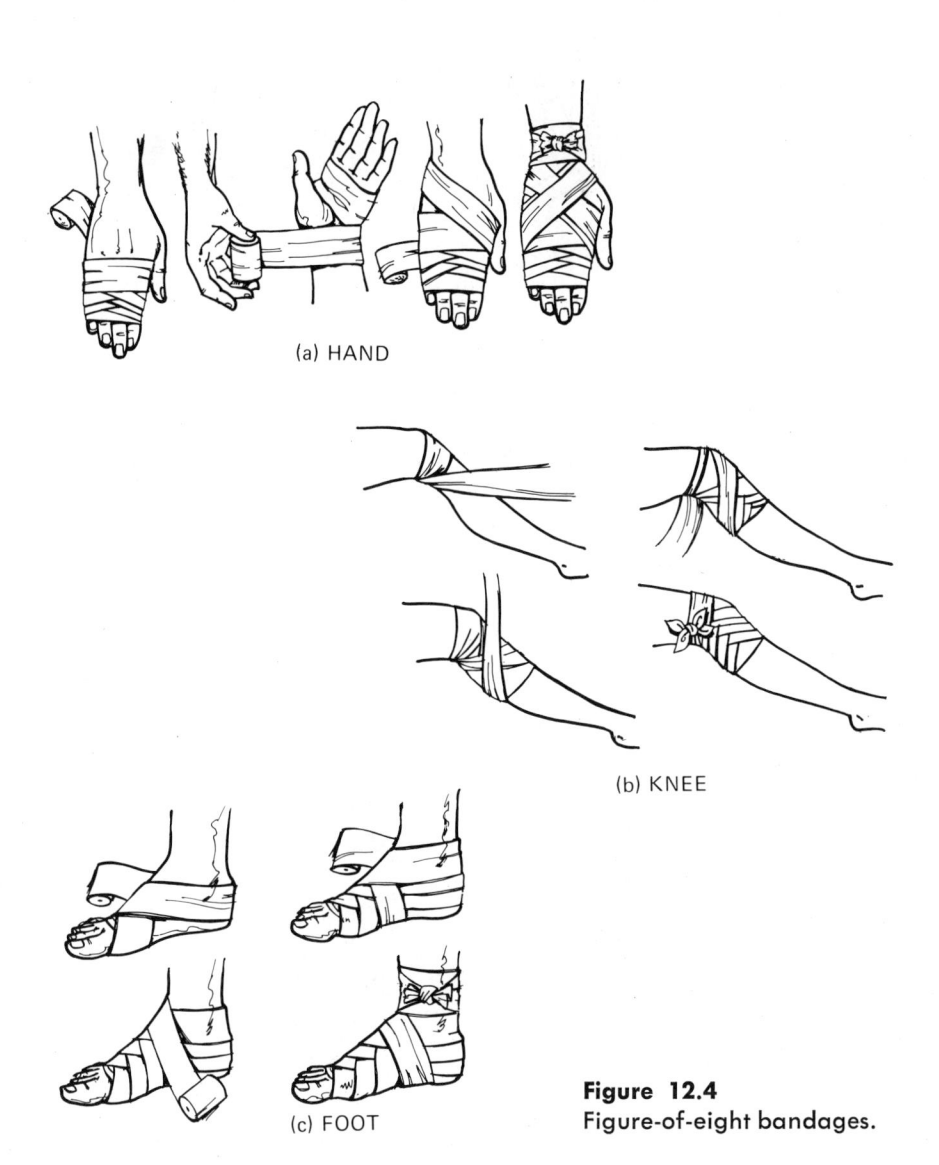

narrow (one-inch) roller gauze and, after applying a sterile compress, unroll gauze from the base of the finger up over the tip and down the other side to the base. After applying several layers of these recurrent turns, closed spiral turns should be applied from the base of the finger to the tip and then back to the base, where it is secured (Figure 12.5).

In applying the *recurrent head bandage* the first aider should apply sterile dressings to the scalp wound and then anchor the roller gauze by making several turns around the head from the forehead above the top of the ears to the back of the head. Complete the last turn at the back of the head and begin a lay from this point across the top of the head to the center of the forehead (Figures 12.6a–b). Continue by adding addi-

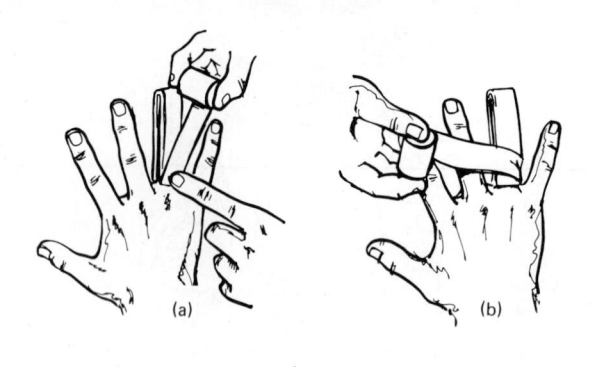

Figure 12.5 Recurrent finger bandage.

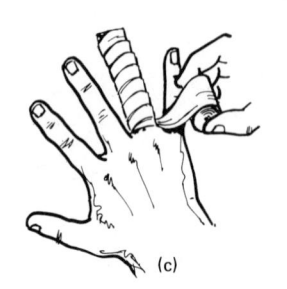

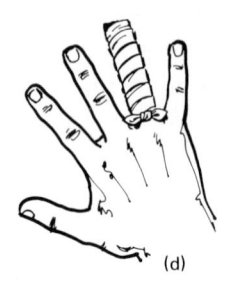

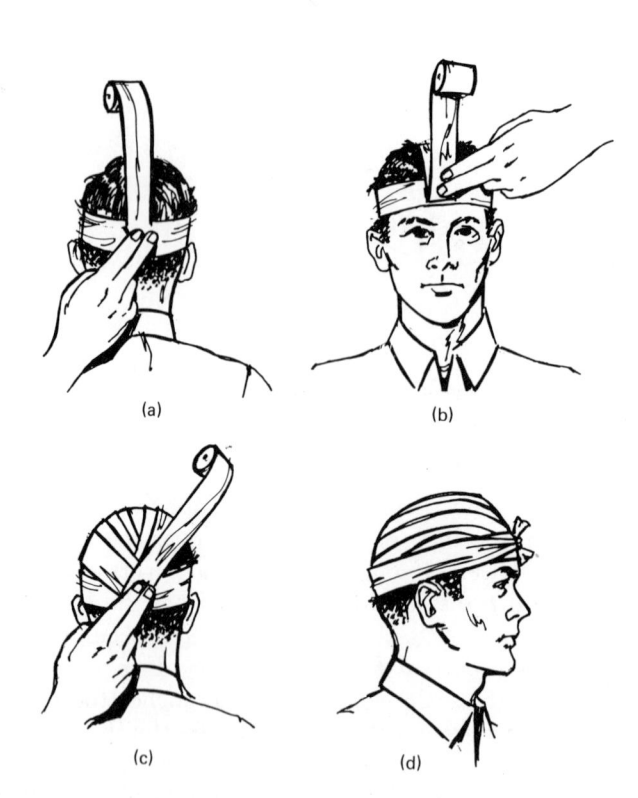

Figure 12.6 Recurrent head bandage.

[184]

tional lays of gauze back to the point at the back of the head, overlapping about half the width of the gauze either to the left or right of the center lay (Figure 12.6c). This back and forth application of the gauze is continued in a recurrent manner until the entire head is covered (Figure 12.6d). The bandage should be secured by making several turns around the head in the same manner that it was anchored and tying or taping it off.

Securing the Bandage

After the bandage has been completely applied, the final step is to secure it in place. This can be done by taping down the end with adhesive tape, pinning with a safety pin, or tying off the end. The easiest method of tying consists of cutting lengthwise into the end of the roller bandage and tying a square knot at the tear. The two ends can then be wrapped in opposite directions around the area being bandaged and tied off to form a secure bandage (Figure 12.7).

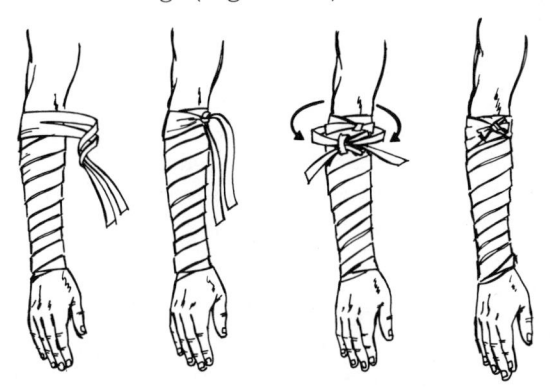

Figure 12.7 Securing the roller gauze by tying off.

Triangular Bandages

Triangular bandages are multi-purpose bandages which may be used in the form of a triangle or folded as a cravat. In the form of a triangle it is useful for bandaging large surfaces such as the scalp or torso, and probably most useful as a sling. In the form of a cravat it can be used instead of a roller gauze and to hold splints in place. Figure 12.8 illustrates the steps for converting a triangular bandage into a cravat.

Application of Triangular Bandages

The *triangular bandage for the head* can be applied much quicker and with less trouble than the recurrent head bandage. The first aider

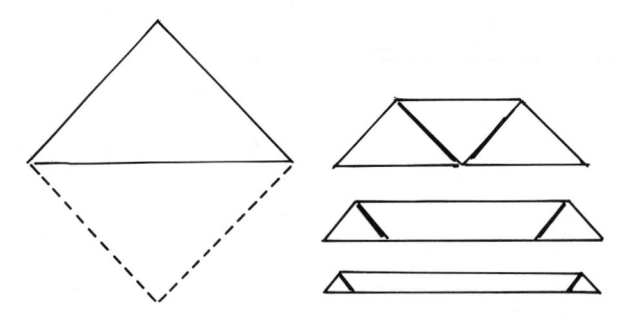

Figure 12.8 Folding a triangular bandage into a cravat.

begins by folding over the long edge of the bandage a couple of times to form approximately two inches of border. Next, the entire bandage is placed flat on the injured individual's head, with the folded border overlapping the forehead (Figure 12.9a). The two ends extending off to the sides of the head are drawn back behind the head where they cross and continue around just above the ears to the center of the forehead (Figures 12.9b–c). The ends should be tied in a square knot. The remaining tail at the back of the head can be tucked over the border for a neater appearance (Figure 12.9d).

A *triangular bandage for the torso* may easily be applied to cover large surfaces such as the chest or back. The first aider should place the right-angled end of the triangle over the shoulder with the large surface of the triangle covering either the back or chest as desired (Figure 12.10a). The

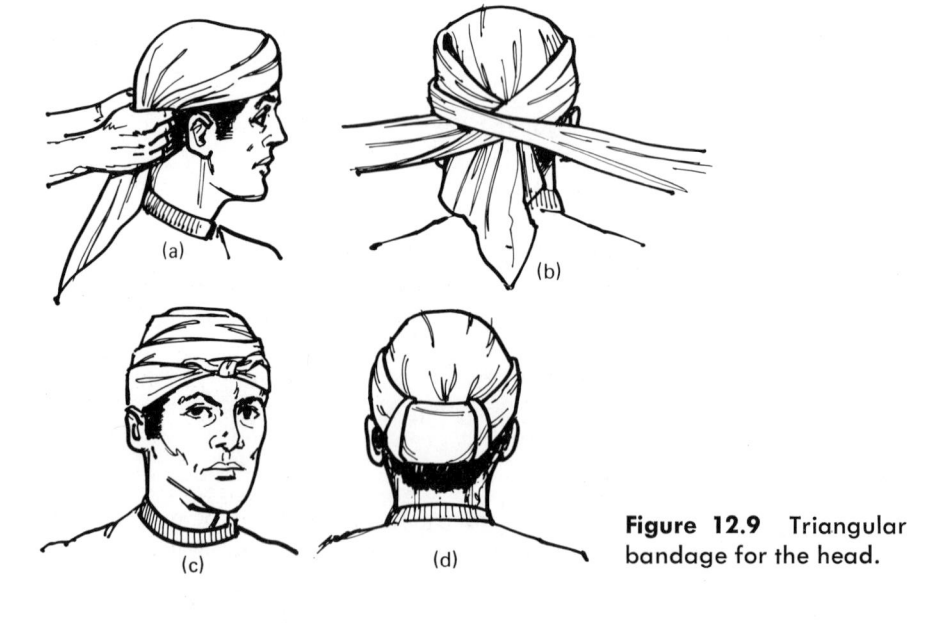

Figure 12.9 Triangular bandage for the head.

remaining two ends are brought around the torso and tied off on the opposite side with the third end (Figures 12.10b–c).

The *cravat bandage for the head* is an easy bandage to apply to head injuries. First the wound is covered with a sterile dressing, then the center of the cravat is placed over the dressing. Each end of the cravat can then be wrapped around the head and snugly tied off in a square knot (Figure 12.11).

The *cravat bandage for the jaw* is a practical bandage for applying dressings in areas of the head, face, and chin. The first aider places a

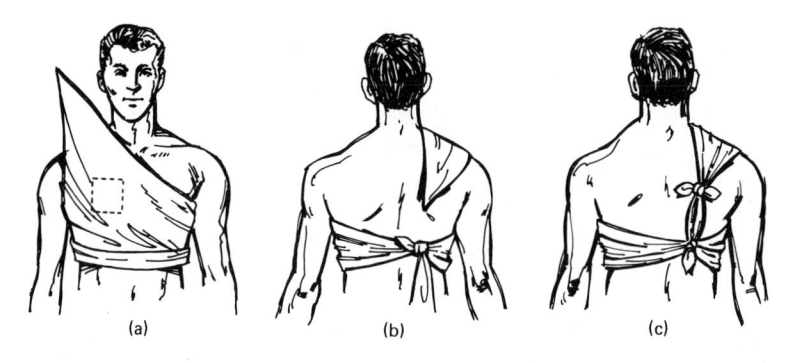

Figure 12.10 Triangular bandage for the torso.

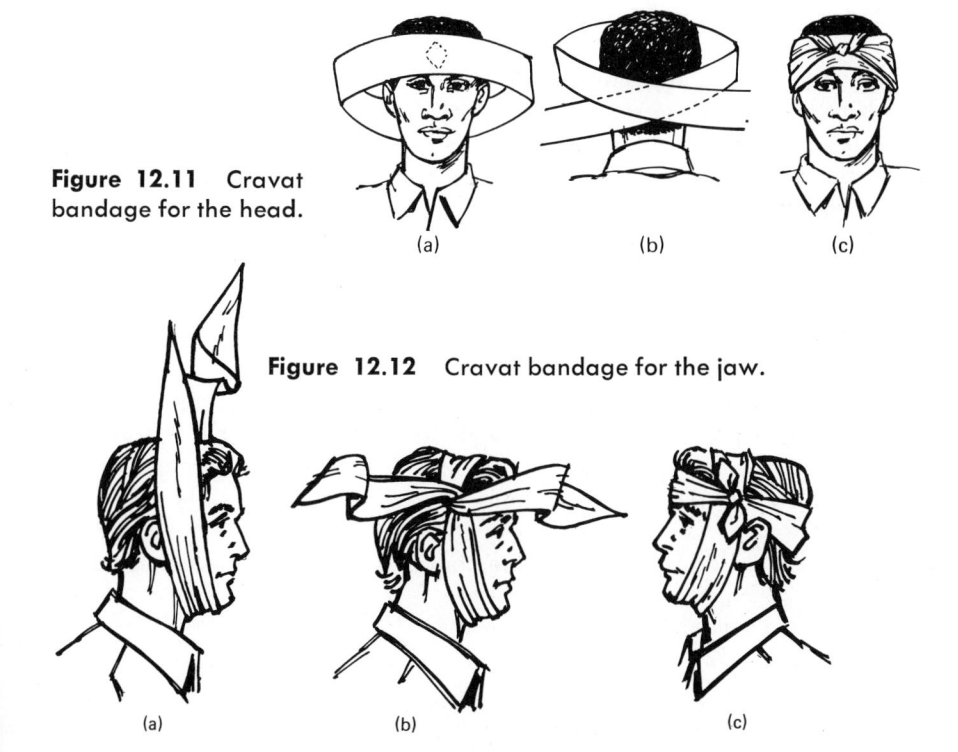

Figure 12.11 Cravat bandage for the head.

Figure 12.12 Cravat bandage for the jaw.

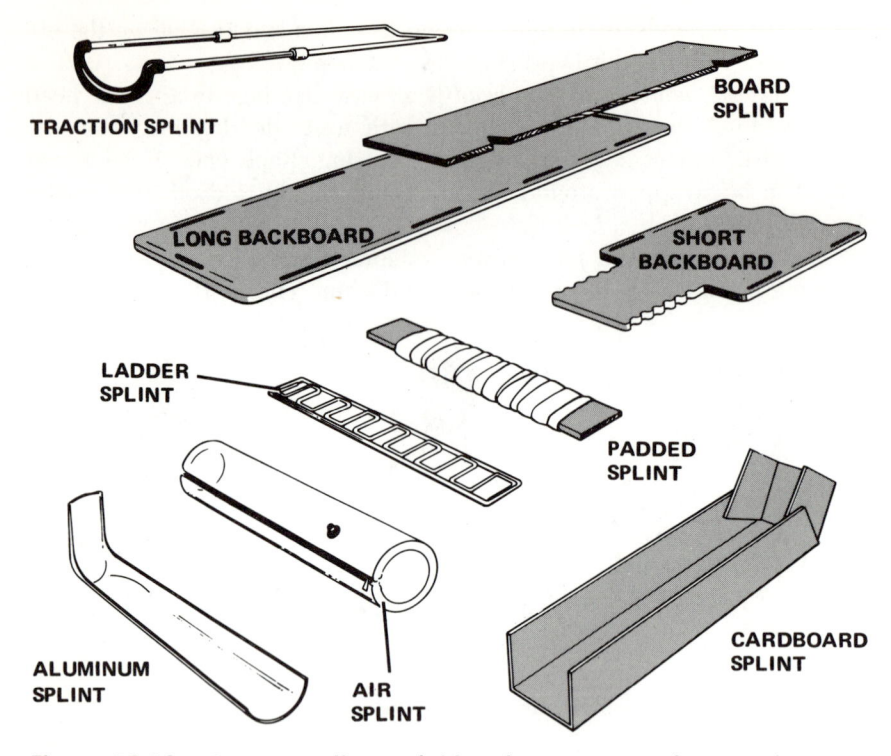

Figure 12.13 Commercially available splinting materials.

cravat under the injured individual's chin, allowing one end to be longer than the other (Figure 12.12a). The two ends are brought up along the side of the face and the longer end is brought over the head to the opposite side (Figure 12.12b). Here the two ends should be crossed and continued around the sides of the head and tied off at the opposite side (Figure 12.12c).

SPLINTING

The importance of splinting fractures or suspected fractures to prevent further injury was discussed in Chapter 6. Reference to that chapter will be helpful in following this discussion.* This section illustrates the various types of splints and methods of applying them to the suspected fractures.

Splints are devices used to immobilize fractures in the legs, arms, or

---

*See also Appendix A, The Skeletal System.

other parts of the body in order to prevent further injury and help reduce pain and shock. Splints may be either the fixation type or the traction type. Fixation splints are used to immobilize the fractured bone ends and adjacent joints through the use of boards of commercially made splints (Figure 12.13). Improvised items that can be used for fixation splints include newspapers and magazines, cardboard, a pillow, umbrella, and so on (Figure 12.14). Fixation splints are relatively easy to apply, and with a little practice the first aider should be able to master the skills of applying this type of splint. Traction splinting is used only on the femur (thigh bone) and requires special handling. A traction splint should be applied by professionally trained individuals.

Application of Fixation Splints

Wrist or Forearm Fracture

1. Use two well-padded splints* that are long enough to extend from the elbow to beyond the finger tips.
2. One splint should be applied so that the palm rests flat against the splint and the other splint along the top of the forearm.
3. The splints should be secured firmly in place using roller gauze or cravat bandages (Figure 12.15a).

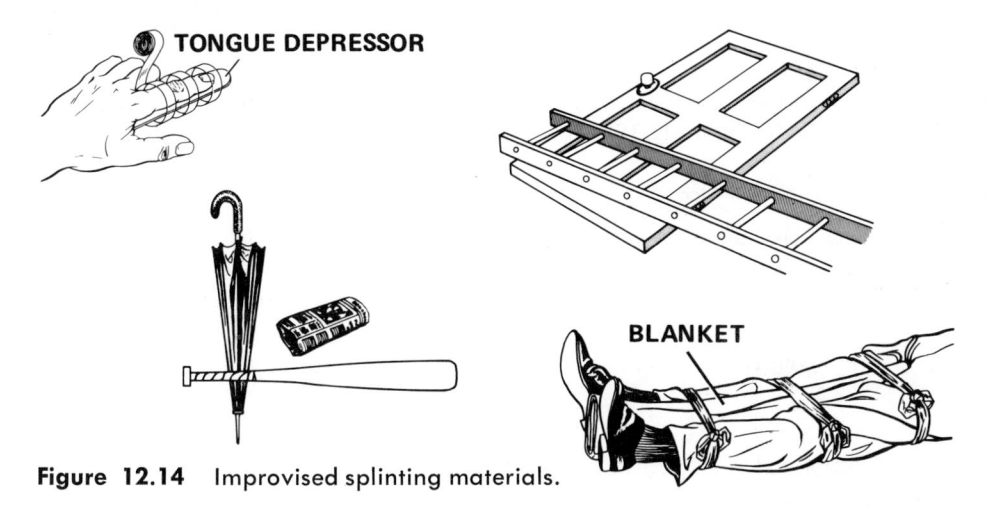

Figure 12.14 Improvised splinting materials.

4. The splinted forearm should be placed in a sling made from a triangular bandage, with the palm resting flat against the chest (Figures 12.15b–c).

*The side of the splint that is placed against the body should be padded with any available soft material such as clothing, towels, or foam rubber.

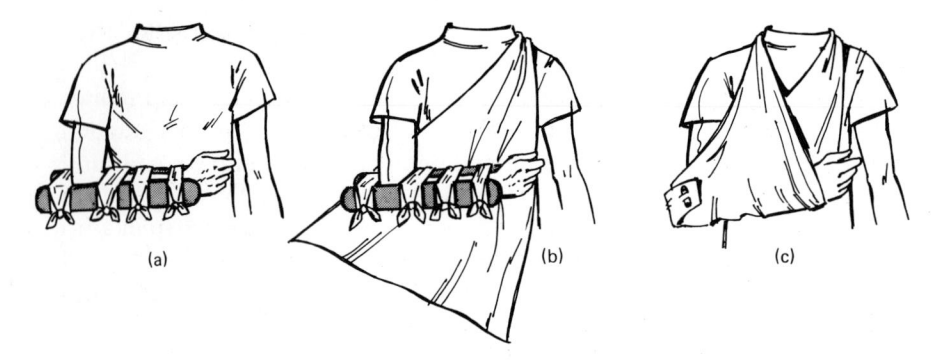

Figure 12.15 Wrist or forearm fixation splint and sling.

Humerus Fracture

1. Use two well-padded splints. One should be long enough to extend from the armpit to below the elbow and the other from the shoulder to below the elbow.
2. One splint should be applied so that it extends from the armpit to just below the elbow. The other should extend on the opposite side of the arm from the shoulder to beyond the elbow. Take care that the end of the splint does not press against the armpit causing a compression of blood vessels.
3. The splints should be secured firmly in place by means of roller gauze or cravat bandages.
4. The splinted area should be placed in a sling as described above (Figure 12.16a).
5. If the fracture is near the shoulder, the first aider should apply padding (such as a folded towel) in the armpit area and bind the arm against the body (Figure 12.16b).

Clavicle Fracture

1. Place the arm on the injured side in a sling with the arm slightly elevated.
2. Secure the arm against the body with a cravat (Figure 12.17).

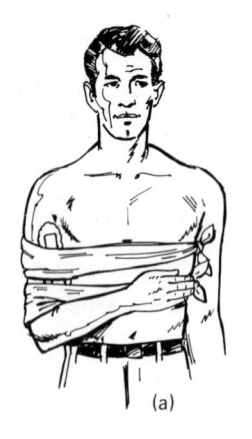

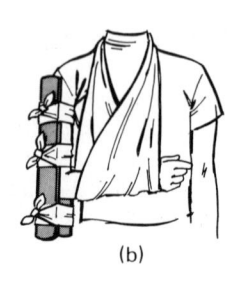

Figure 12.16 Humerus fixation splint.

First Aid Practical Skills   [191]

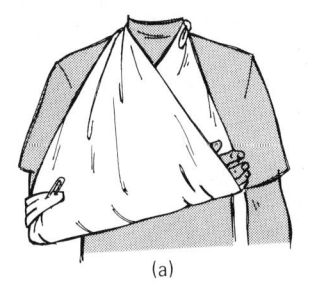

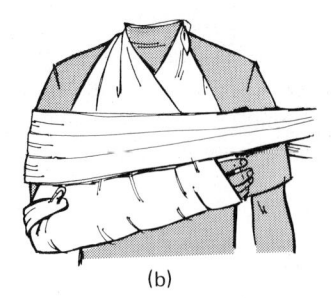

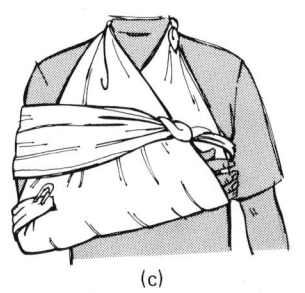

Figure 12.17 Clavicle fixation splint.

Elbow Fracture

1. If the arm is fully extended, use two well-padded splints long enough to extend from the armpit to beyond the finger tips and from shoulder to beyond the finger tips.
2. One splint should be applied so that it extends from the armpit to just beyond the finger tips. The other splint should extend on the opposite side of the arm from the shoulder to the finger tips (Figure 12.18a).

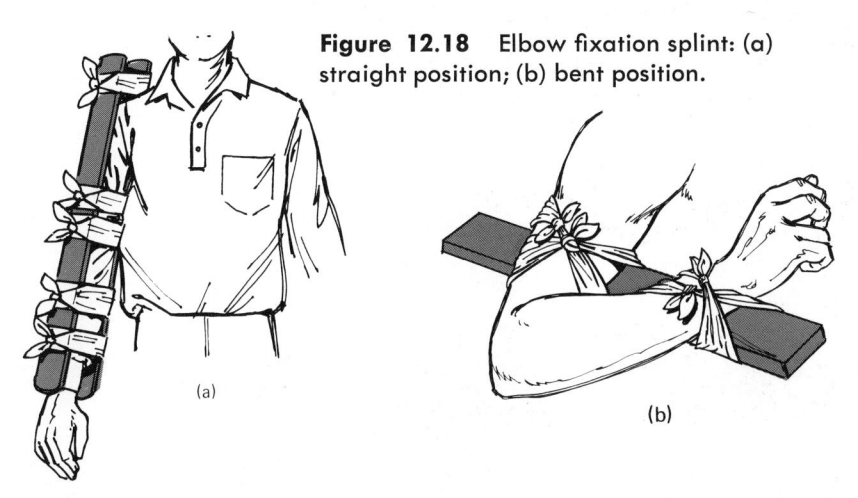

Figure 12.18 Elbow fixation splint: (a) straight position; (b) bent position.

3. The splints should be secured firmly in place with the use of roller gauze or cravat bandages.
4. If the arm is found bent at the elbow, it must be splinted in the position as found. *No attempt should be made to straighten the arm.* In this situation one splint may be used, as illustrated in Figure 12.18b. If two splints are used, the second is applied over the first, with the bent arm secured between the two splints as discussed above.

Finger Fracture

1. Apply a tongue depressor or other rigid material to the underside of the finger.
2. Secure with roller gauze using an open spiral bandage or strips of adhesive tape (Figure 12.19).

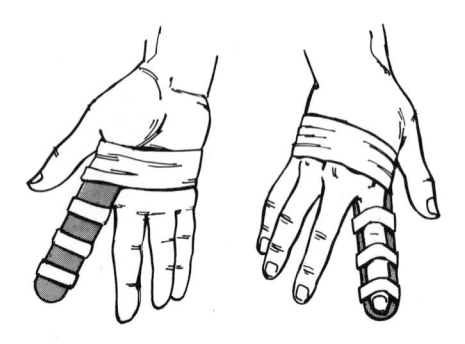

Figure 12.19 Finger fixation splint.

Femur Fracture

1. Use two well-padded splints. One splint should be long enough to extend from the armpit to at least six inches beyond the heel and the other from the groin to at least six inches beyond the heel.
2. Apply the splints on each side of the leg, one from the groin to the heel

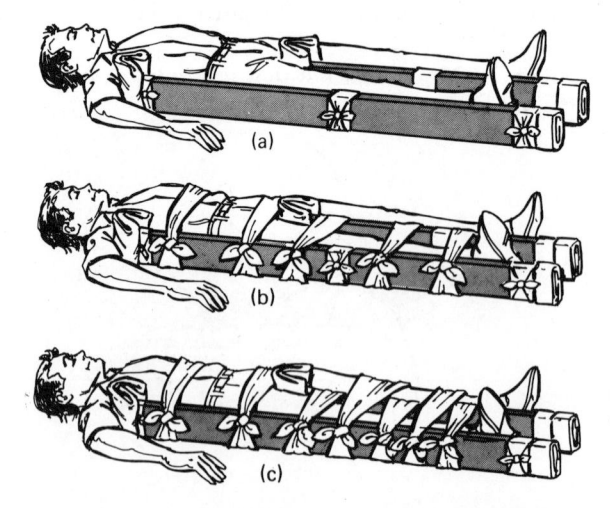

Figure 12.20 Femur fixation splint.

and the other from the armpit to the heel. The ends of the splints should be padded (Figure 12.20a).
3. Use several cravats to secure the two splints to the injured leg between the groin and ankle (Figure 12.20b). Then apply several more cravats securing the longer splint to the torso and the other leg (Figure 12.20c).

Lower Leg Fracture

1. Use two well-padded splints of equal length. The splints should be long enough to extend from the groin to the heel.
2. Apply the splints on each side of the leg, one from the groin to the heel and the other on the outside of the leg opposite the first splint.
3. Use several cravats to secure the splints to the leg (Figure 12.21).

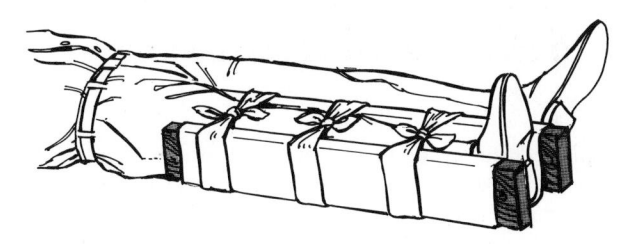

Figure 12.21 Lower leg fixation splint.

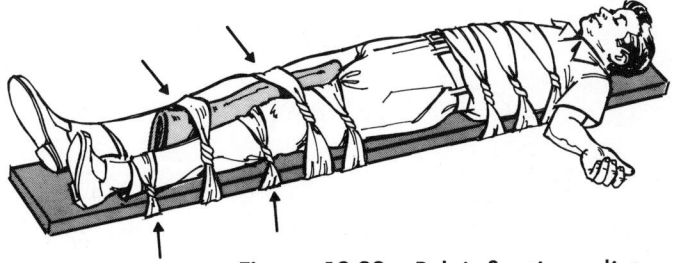

Figure 12.22 Pelvis fixation splint.

Pelvic Fracture

1. Use a long wooden splint that is at least six inches wide and longer than the entire length of the injured individual. A commercial backboard is ideal for this type of injury.
2. The injured individual should be carefully placed on the splint, lying on his back.
3. Place a folded blanket between the legs to act as padding.
4. Secure the leg on the injured side of the body to the splint, using several cravats. Also secure the uninjured leg to the splint for further stability (Figure 12.22).

Patella (Knee) Fracture

1. If the knee is found in a straight position, use one padded splint that is long enough to extend from the buttocks to beyond the heel.
2. The splint should be applied under the leg with extra padding provided under the knee and ankle. Secure the splint to the leg with several cravats (Figure 12.23).
3. If the leg is found in a bent position *no attempt should be made to straighten it.* Splint in the bent position using the same technique as for an elbow fracture.

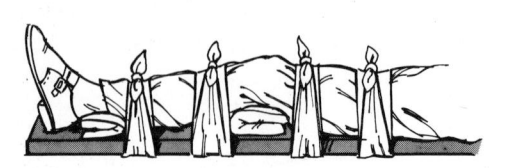

Figure 12.23 Patella fixation splint.

Rib Fracture

1. Rib fractures are splinted simply by tying three cravats around the injured individual's chest. Place the first cravat in the center of the chest, tighten it as the individual exhales, and secure it by tying a square knot on the uninjured side (Figure 12.24a). An additional cravat should be placed above and below the first one, as in (b) and (c).
2. Padding should be placed under the knots as they are being tied on the uninjured side.

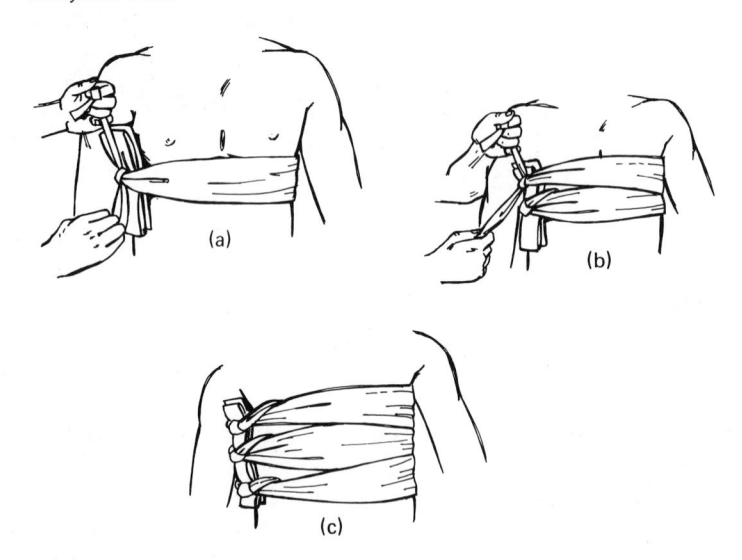

Figure 12.24 Rib fixation splint.

First Aid Practical Skills   [195]

Spinal Fractures—Full Backboard

1. A full backboard must be used whenever a back or neck fracture or injury is suspected.
2. At least four people are needed to place the injured individual on the backboard so as not to cause further injury.
3. The backboard is placed parallel to and alongside the injured individual. Three first aiders should place themselves in a kneeling position along the opposite side of the injured individual (Figure 12.25a). The fourth first aider should position himself at the head the injured individual. He

(a)

(b)

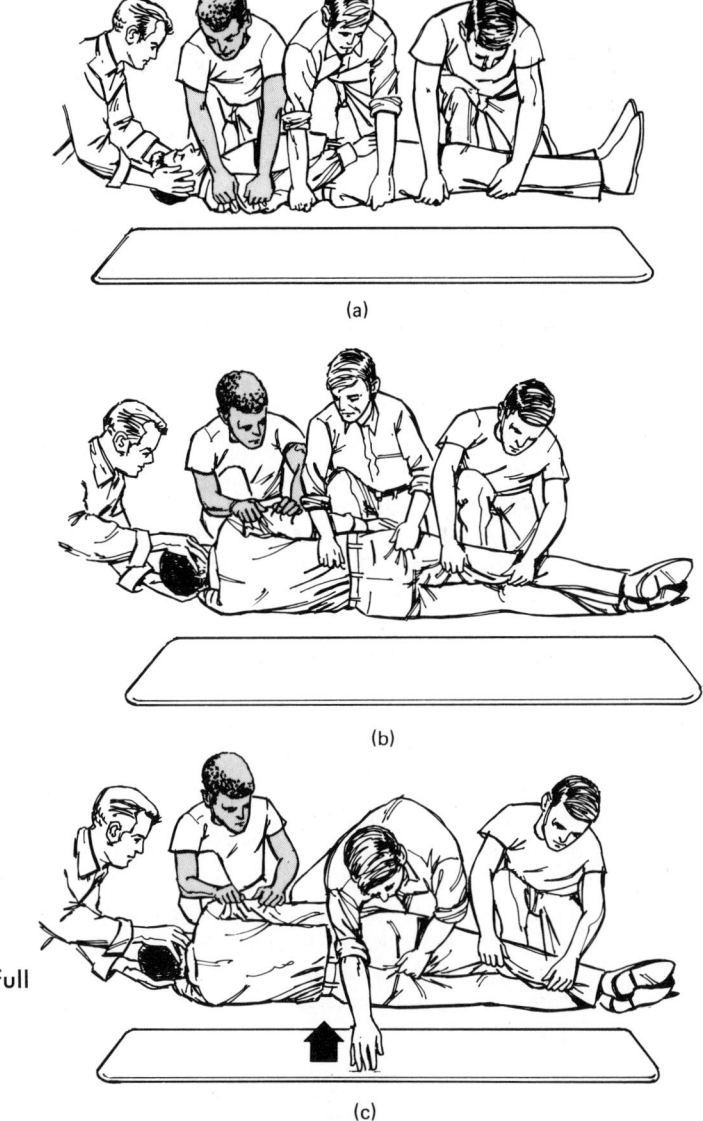

Figure 12.25
Application of a full backboard.

(c)

[196] First Aid Practical Skills

(d)

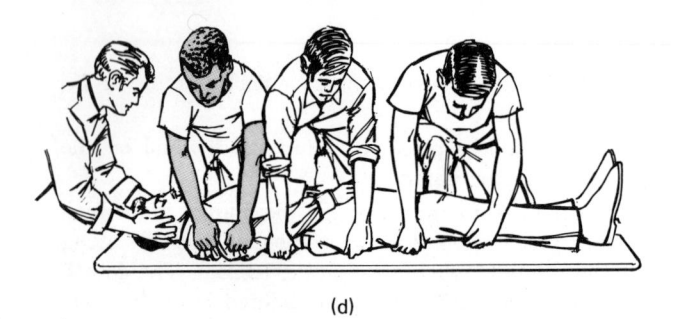

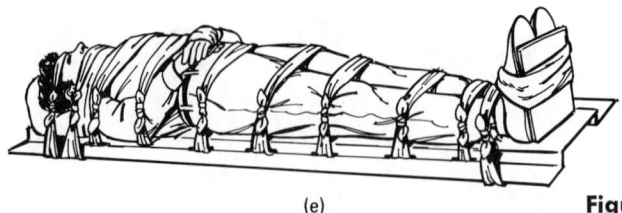

(e)   Figure 12.25 (continued)

must hold the head securely in his hands at the same time as the body is being moved.

4. The object is for the first aiders to support the various parts of the individual's body while he is rolled in their direction (Figure 12.25b). The center first aider slides the backboard under the injured individual (Figure 12.25c) and then the injured individual is gently rolled back onto the backboard (Figure 12.25d). This entire operation requires a great deal of coordination, and one first aider, preferably the one holding the head, should give the commands for moving.

5. Once the injured individual is on the backboard his head must be secured with a blanket roll or by some other means to insure immobility. The rest of the body should be tied to the backboard with cravats (Figure 12.25e).

Spinal Fractures—Half Backboard

1. The half backboard is used in situations where the full backboard cannot easily be maneuvered into position, for example, an injured individual found in a sitting position in an automobile collision. The half backboard is not to be used for carrying an individual, and must be used in conjunction with a full backboard.

2. One first aider positions himself behind the injured individual and supports the head by applying slight upward traction (Figure 12.26a). The other first aider slips the half backboard behind the individual's back and as far down below the pelvic region as possible (Figure 12.26b).

3. Any voids, such as behind the curvature of the neck, should be padded to insure complete immobilization. A cervical collar or blanket roll should

First Aid Practical Skills [197]

be applied to prevent any head motion. The head should be secured to the board by tying a cravat bandage around the forehead and another around the collar to the board. Straps or long cravats should be placed around the individual's chest and waist to secure him to the backboard (Figure 12.26c).

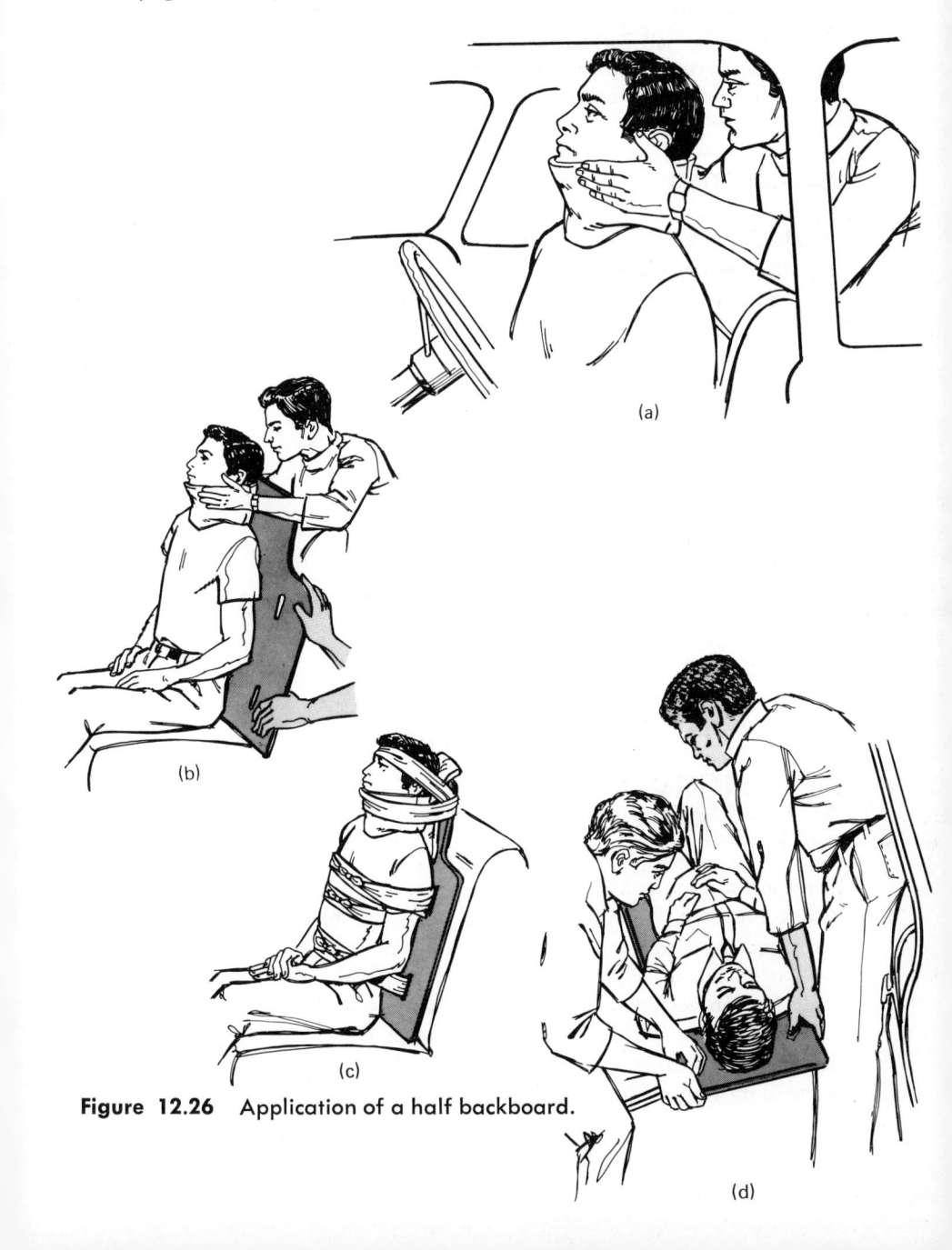

Figure 12.26 Application of a half backboard.

[198] First Aid Practical Skills

4. The splinted individual is now ready to be placed on the full backboard. He should slowly be turned and placed in a reclining position as he is being slid onto the full backboard (Figure 12.26d). The first aider must fully support the injured individual's body during this operation. No attempt should be made to lift him by pulling on the half backboard as it may slip and the neck would move causing further injury.
5. Once the half backboard is placed onto the full backboard and extrication is completed, the injured individual should be secured to the full backboard with cravats to prevent any further body movement.

TRANSPORTING

There are very few times when any attempt should be made to move a badly injured individual. It is always best to administer life-saving first aid and await the professional assistance of an ambulance crew or rescue squad to extricate the injured individual. In cases of back, neck, or head injuries, internal injuries, or severe fractures, improper movement or

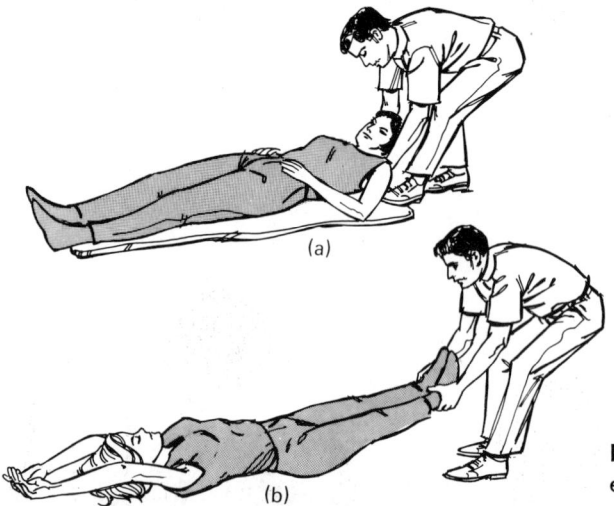

Figure 12.27 One-man emergency transfer.

transportation may aggravate the injuries or even cause death. There are times, however, when an individual will have to be moved because the surrounding dangers may be potentially more serious than the injuries he has sustained. Examples include an injured individual in a burning building, an accident victim lying in a puddle of gasoline or on a busy highway, or an individual who may be in danger from a building collapse. In such cases, where there is immediate danger, the first aider will have to move quickly and decisively. It is best to drag an injured individual to safety by his shoulders in the direction of the long axis of the body (Figure 12.27a). This is especially important if the individual has suffered a back injury or leg fracture. Any motion from the sides or twisting of the torso could aggravate or increase the existing injury and even cause permanent damage. If the shoulders are inaccessible, it may be necessary to drag the individual by his feet (Figure 12.27b). This procedure, is not recommended, however, unless absolutely necessary.

There are numerous methods by which a person can be moved or transported, but only the more common, less complicated methods will be described here. The first aider must remember that under varying emergency situations some of these methods may not work, and he will have to improvise, as is so often the case when giving emergency first aid.

Two-Man Carry

The two-man carry can be used if the injured individual is conscious and has sustained only minor injuries. The two first aiders interlock two arms as shown in Figure 12.28a. The injured individual sits on their arms while the first aiders' other two arms are used to support his back (Figure 12.28b). The injured individual helps to support himself by placing his arms around the shoulders of the first aiders (Figures 12.28c–d). He is then ready to be lifted and carried to safety.

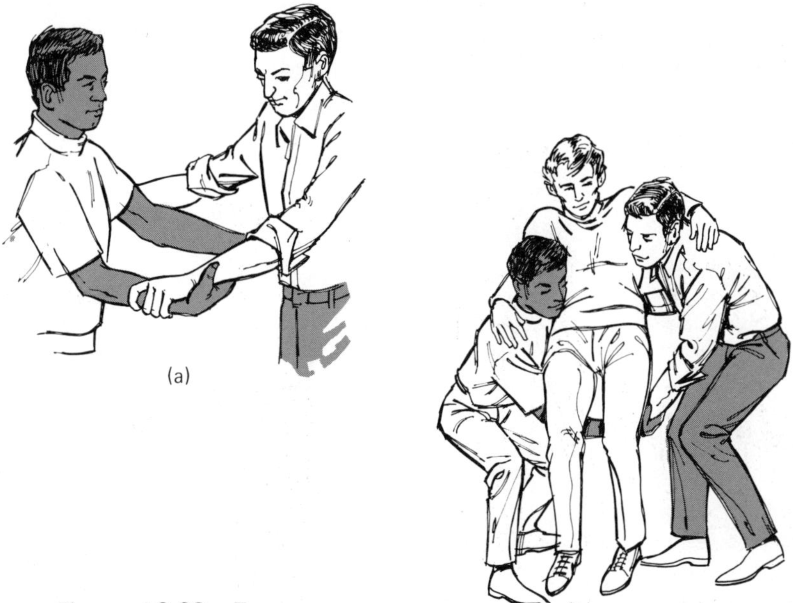

Figure 12.28 Two-man carry.

(c)

(d)

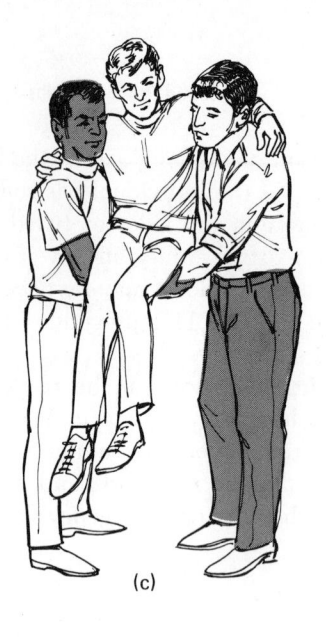

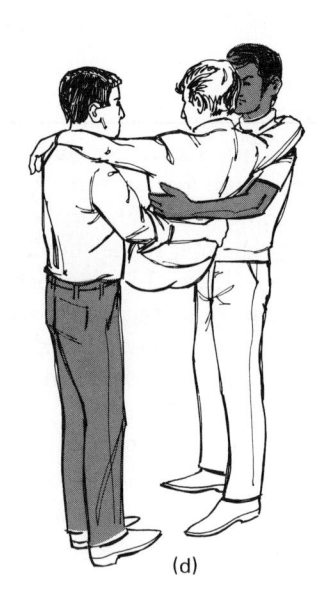

Chair Carry

The chair carry is especially helpful when moving an injured person up or down stairways or from rooms that require maneuvering around sharp corners or through narrow hallways. The injured individual is placed on a sturdy, four-legged chair. Never use a folding, swivel, single-pedestal, or flimsy chair. One first aider holds the back of the chair while the other holds the front legs (Figure 12.29a). As the first aider holding the back of the chair tilts it backward, the first aider in the front lifts up (Figure 12.29b). This carry gives little support to the back or legs and should not be used when these areas are injured.

(a)

(b)

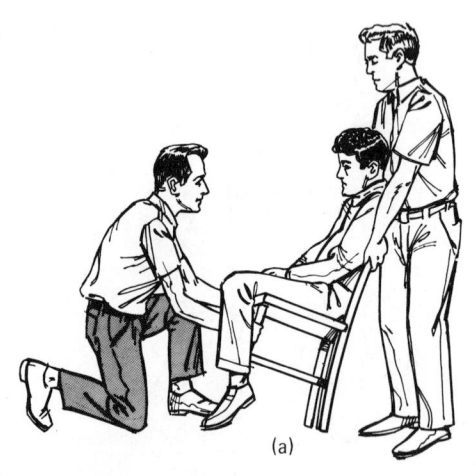

Figure 12.29 Chair carry.

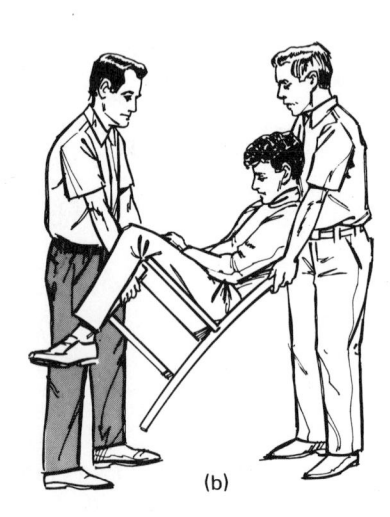

Blanket Lift

Often a blanket can be used as an improvised stretcher to carry an injured individual. A blanket gives poor support so this method of transportation should not be used in cases of back injury. The first step in the blanket lift is to place the individual on the blanket. The first aider should take a long blanket and, holding one of the long ends, allow about two thirds of the blanket to fall in pleats (Figure 12.30a). With the injured individual lying on his back, place the pleated side of the blanket along one side of him. The first aider now kneels along the opposite side of the individual and slowly rolls him towards himself. The pleated portion of the blanket should now be placed as far under the individual as possible (Figure 12.30b). The injured individual is now allowed to slowly roll back onto the blanket, the pleats are pulled out on the first aider's side, and the individual is centered on the blanket (Figure 12.30c).

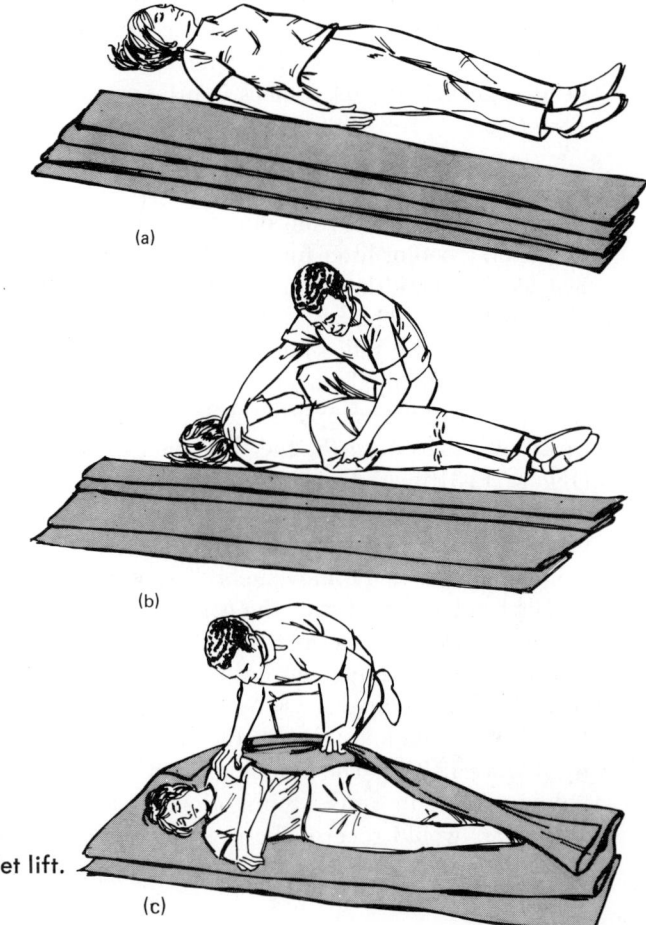

Figure 12.30 Blanket lift.

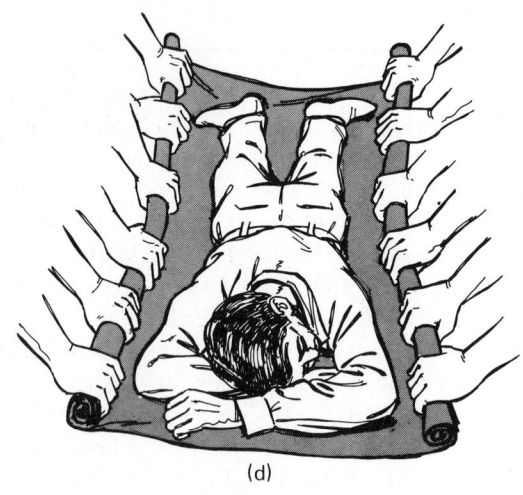

Figure 12.30 (continued)
(d)

It will take six first aiders to hold the blanket securely. The sides of the blanket may be rolled up and used as handles to lift the individual as illustrated in Figure 12.30d. One first aider should support the injured's head, especially if back or neck injuries are suspected.

Three-Man Lift and Carry

The three-man lift from one side is useful for placing an injured individual on a bed or litter for carrying him through a narrow area. All three first aiders should kneel on one knee on the same side of the individual (Figure 12.31a). The first aiders then place their hands under the injured individual in the following manner: (1) The first man places one hand under the individual's neck and the other hand under his upper back; (2) the center man supports the lower back with one hand and the buttocks with the other; (3) the third man places his hands under the legs (Figure 12.31b). As the legs are the lightest in weight, the weakest first aider should be used to support this segment of the body. The first aiders are now ready to lift the individual. The entire lifting action must be completed as a single movement. To insure that everyone lifts in unison, one first aider should give the command to move. The first step is to lift the individual onto the first aiders' bent knees (Figure 12.31c). From this position the individual can be placed on an adjacent ambulance litter or bed. If the individual must be carried, then the first aiders' next step is to roll the individual towards themselves (Figure 12.31d) and then stand up (Figure 12.31e). The first aiders can now transport the injured individual by moving in a side step motion. To lower the injured individual the first aiders would reverse the previous steps, that is, return to the kneeling position, etc.

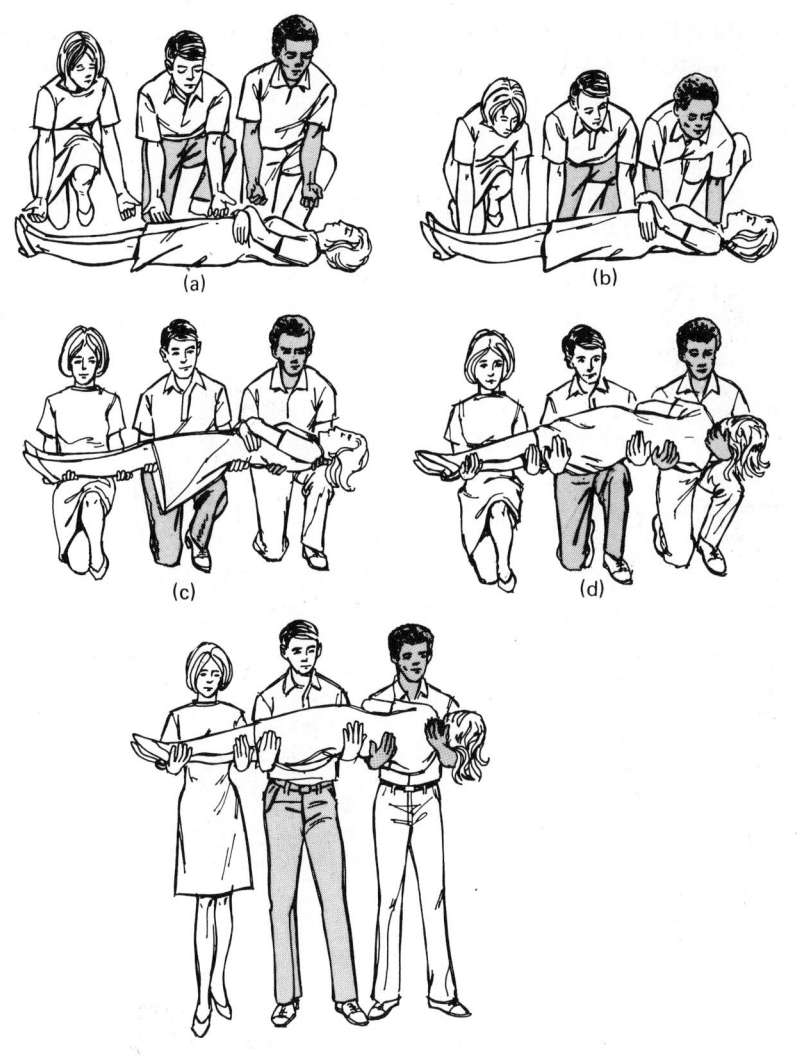

(e) **Figure 12.31** Three-man lift and carry.

Three-Man Hammock Carry

The three-man hammock carry offers several advantages over the three-man lift and carry. With the hammock first aiders can carry the injured individual a longer distance because they can walk in a forward direction. There is also less chance of their feet tripping, since the center first aider is facing the two side first aiders. On the same side of the individual, one first aider kneels at the upper portion of the body while a second first aider kneels at the lower portion. On the opposite side of the body a third first aider kneels at the center portion of the injured individual. The center first aider then interlocks his wrists with the inside hands of the first aiders he is facing (Figure 12.32a). This results in a stronger configuration for lifting the individual. Again, one person must give the command to insure a single movement. Upon command, the first aiders lift the individual to the kneeling position (Figure 12.32b) and then to the standing position (Figure 12.32c).

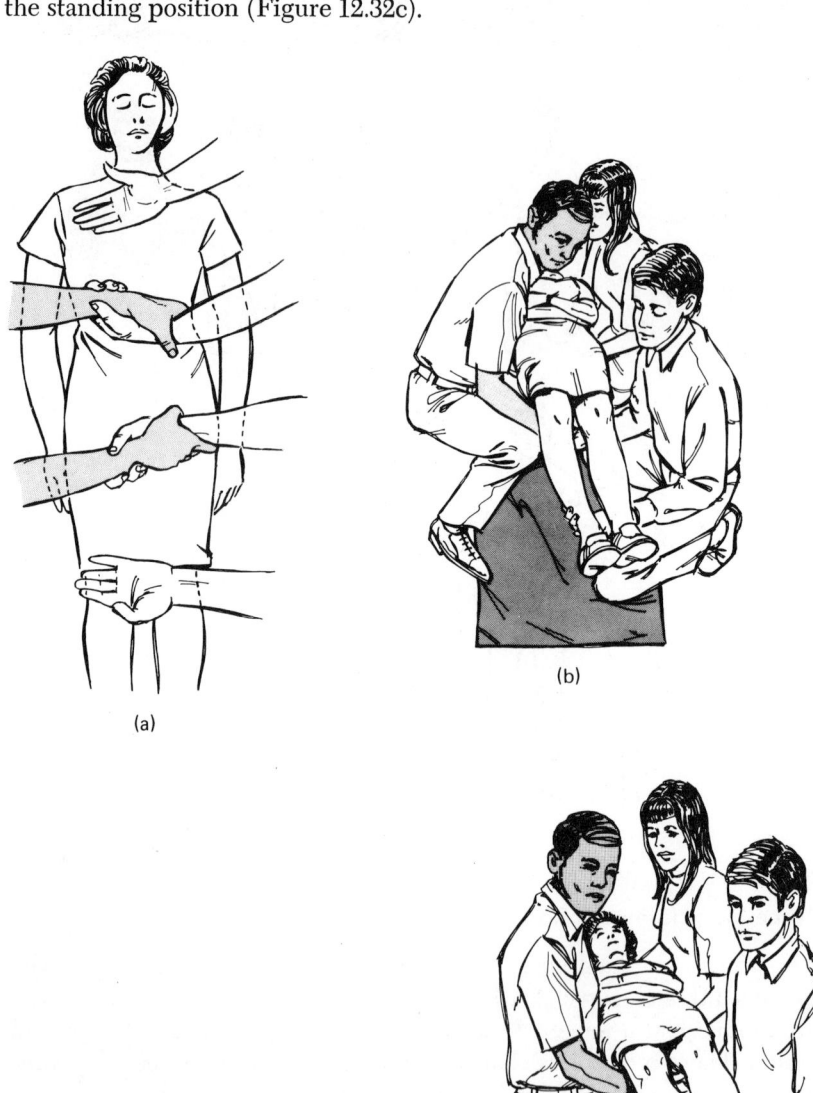

Figure 12.32 Three-man hammock carry.

First Aid Practical Skills   [205]

Six-Man Lift and Carry

The six-man lift and carry is similar to the three-man carry, except that there are more first aiders available thus requiring less lifting power from each person and providing more support to the injured individual. This mode of transport is especially useful when the injured is a heavy individual. Three first aiders place themselves on either side of the individual. Their hands are slipped under the injured individual in an alternating manner and are interlocked for greater support (Figure 12.33a). The indi-

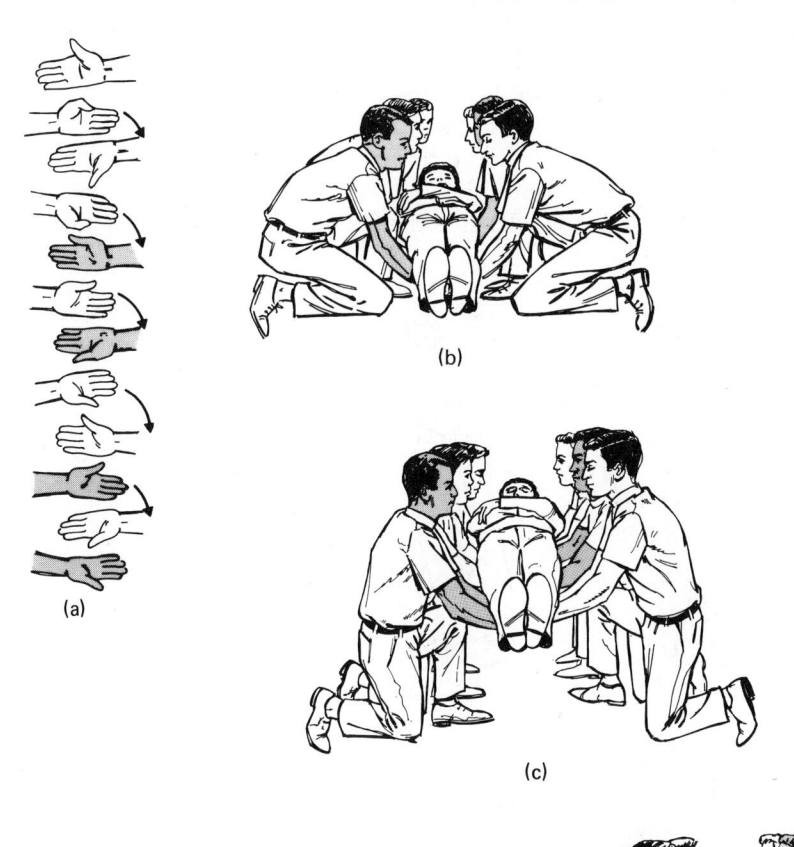

Figure 12.33 Six-man lift and carry.

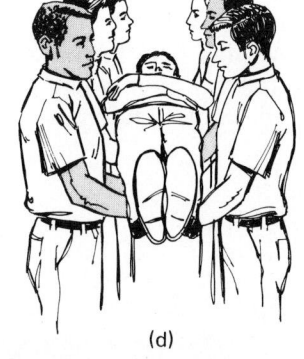

vidual is then lifted upon command as previously described and as shown in Figures 12.33b–d.

As more people are involved in this lift than with the others, the importance of moving in unison is even more important. One first aider must give the commands, and a cooperatiave effort to move in one motion must be made.

Stretcher Carry

A variety of stretchers and litters are available for transporting the injured. Moving an individual by stretcher is a relatively easy matter, the most complicated part usually being the manner in which the individual is placed on or removed from the stretcher. Most of the previously described lifts and carries can be used to place the injured individual on or lift him off a stretcher. Once the injured individual is lying on the stretcher, one first aider should give the "lift" and "forward" commands

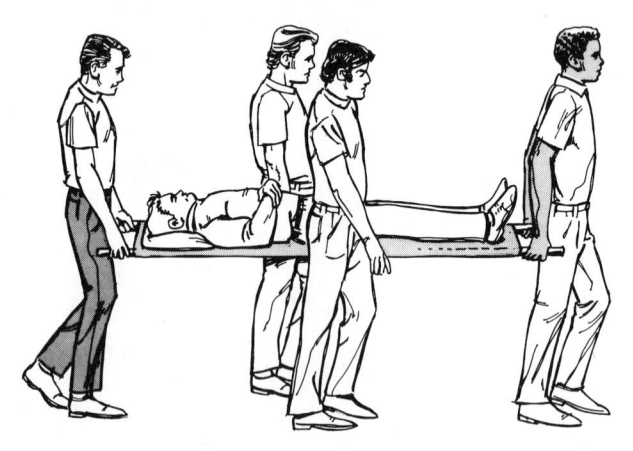

Figure 12.34 Stretcher carry.

so as to insure smooth movement. If two first aiders are lifting the stretcher, they should position themselves at the head and at the foot, facing each other, which means that the first aider at the foot end will be walking backwards. If there are four first aiders available to carry the stretcher, they would position themselves as shown in Figure 12.34, which allows all to face in the same direction of travel.

APPENDIXES

APPENDIXES

Appendix A: THE SKELETAL SYSTEM

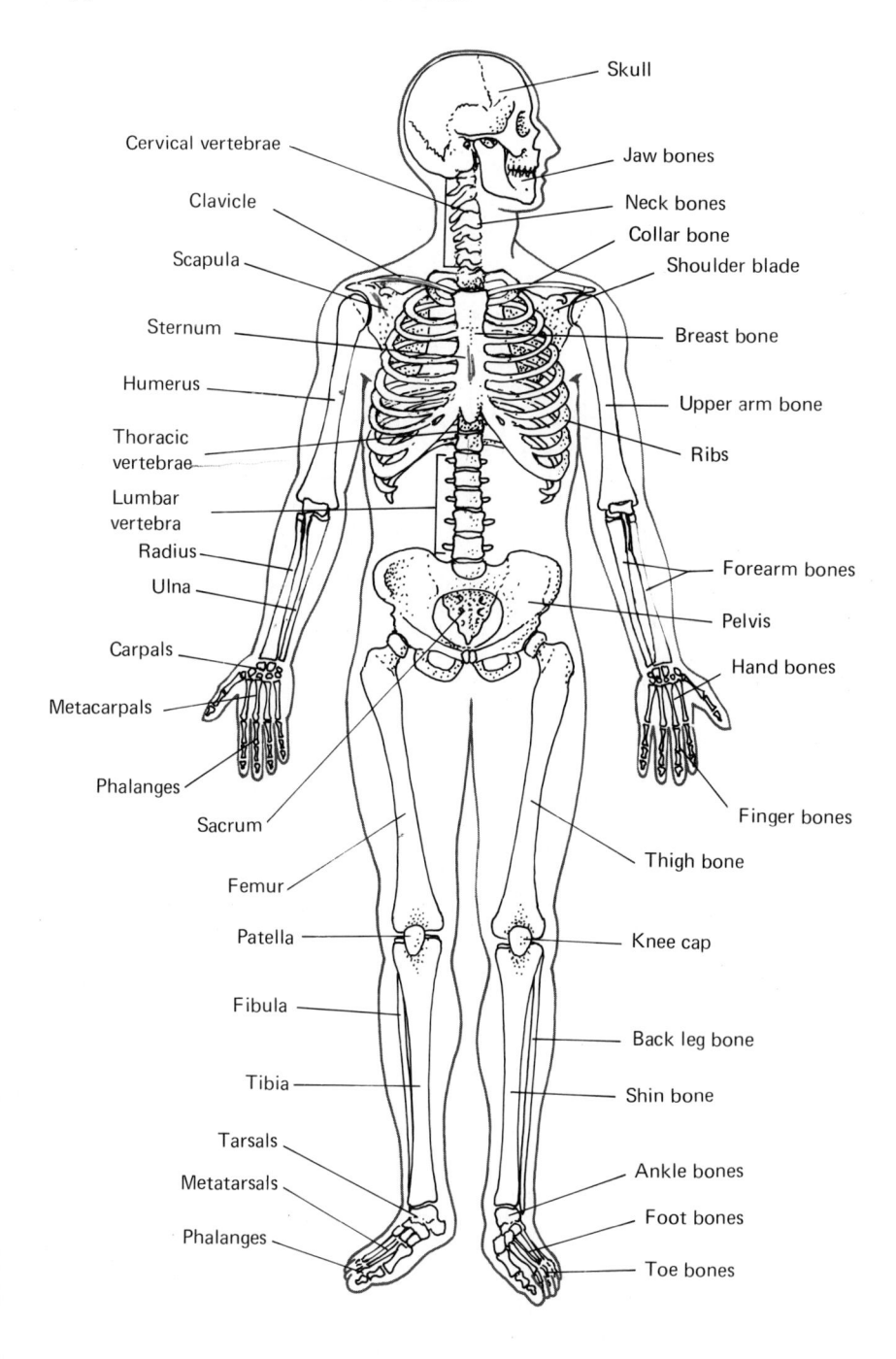

Anatomical name	Common name
Skull	—
Cervical vertebrae	Neck bones
—	Jaw bones
Clavicle	Collar bone
Scapula	Shoulder blade
Sternum	Breast bone
Humerus	Upper arm bone
Thoracic vertebrae	—
—	Ribs
Lumbar vertebra	—
Radius	Forearm bones
Ulna	
Carpals	Hand bones
Metacarpals	
Phalanges	Finger bones
Sacrum	—
Femur	Thigh bone
Patella	Knee cap
Fibula	Back leg bone
Tibia	Shin bone
Tarsals	Ankle bones
Metatarsals	Foot bones
Phalanges	Toe bones

Appendix B: THE HEART

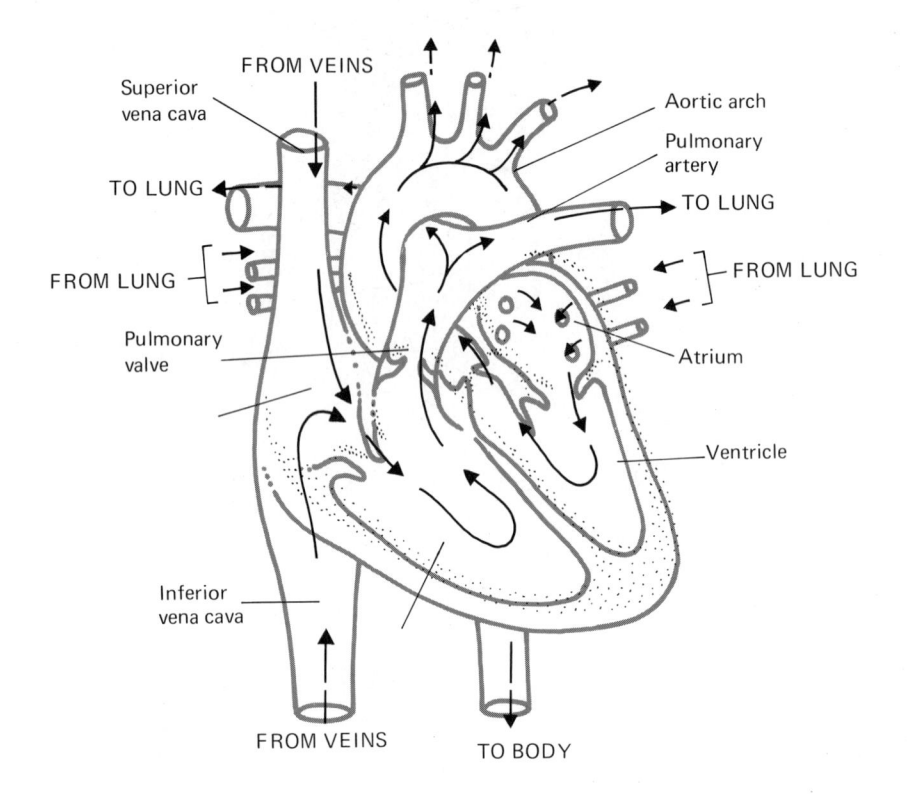

Appendix C: THE CIRCULATORY SYSTEM

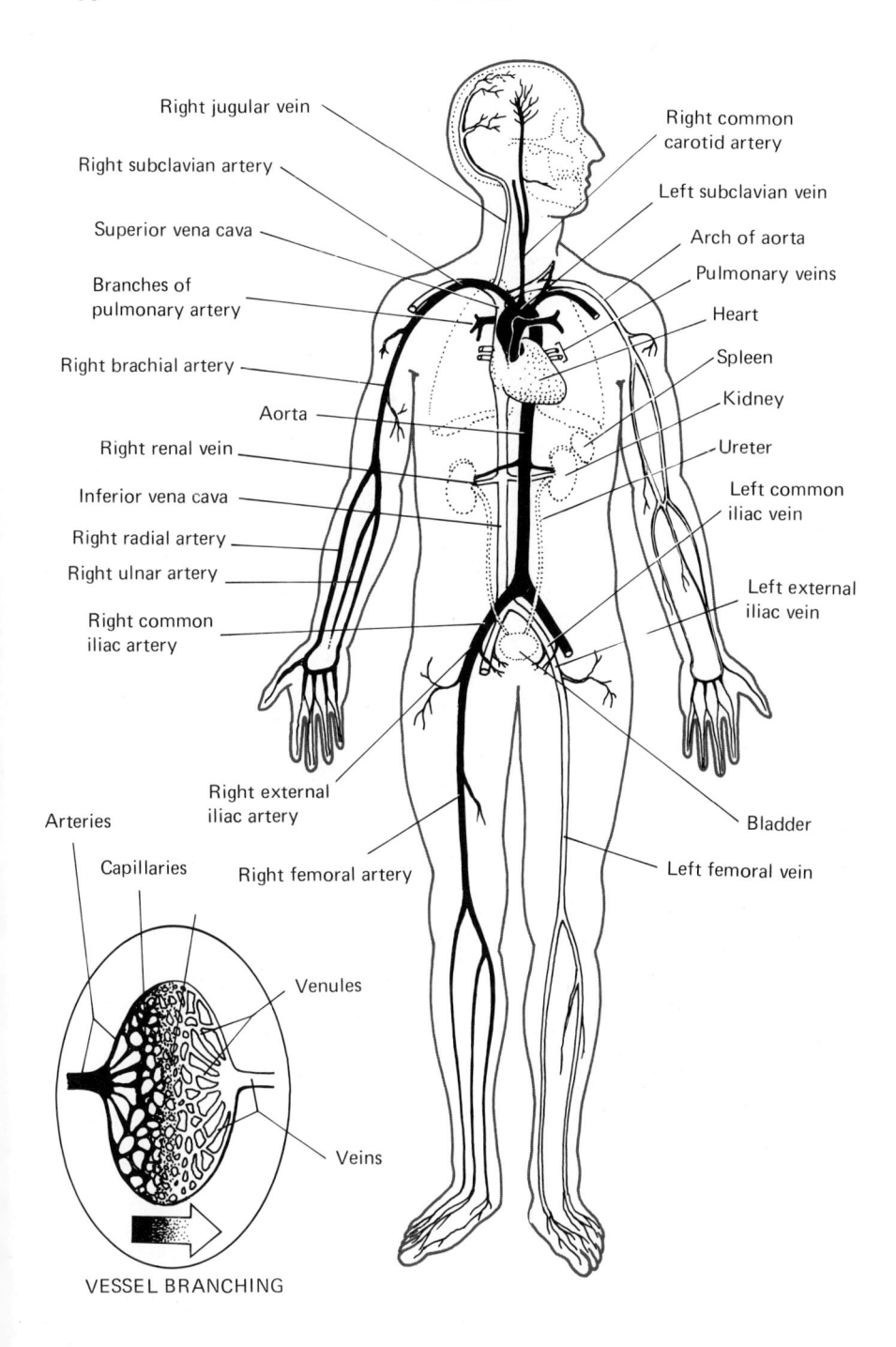

Right jugular vein
Right subclavian artery
Superior vena cava
Branches of pulmonary artery
Right brachial artery
Aorta
Right renal vein
Inferior vena cava
Right radial artery
Right ulnar artery
Right common iliac artery
Right external iliac artery
Right femoral artery

Right common carotid artery
Left subclavian vein
Arch of aorta
Pulmonary veins
Heart
Spleen
Kidney
Ureter
Left common iliac vein
Left external iliac vein
Bladder
Left femoral vein

Arteries
Capillaries
Venules
Veins

VESSEL BRANCHING

211

Appendix D: THE RESPIRATORY SYSTEM

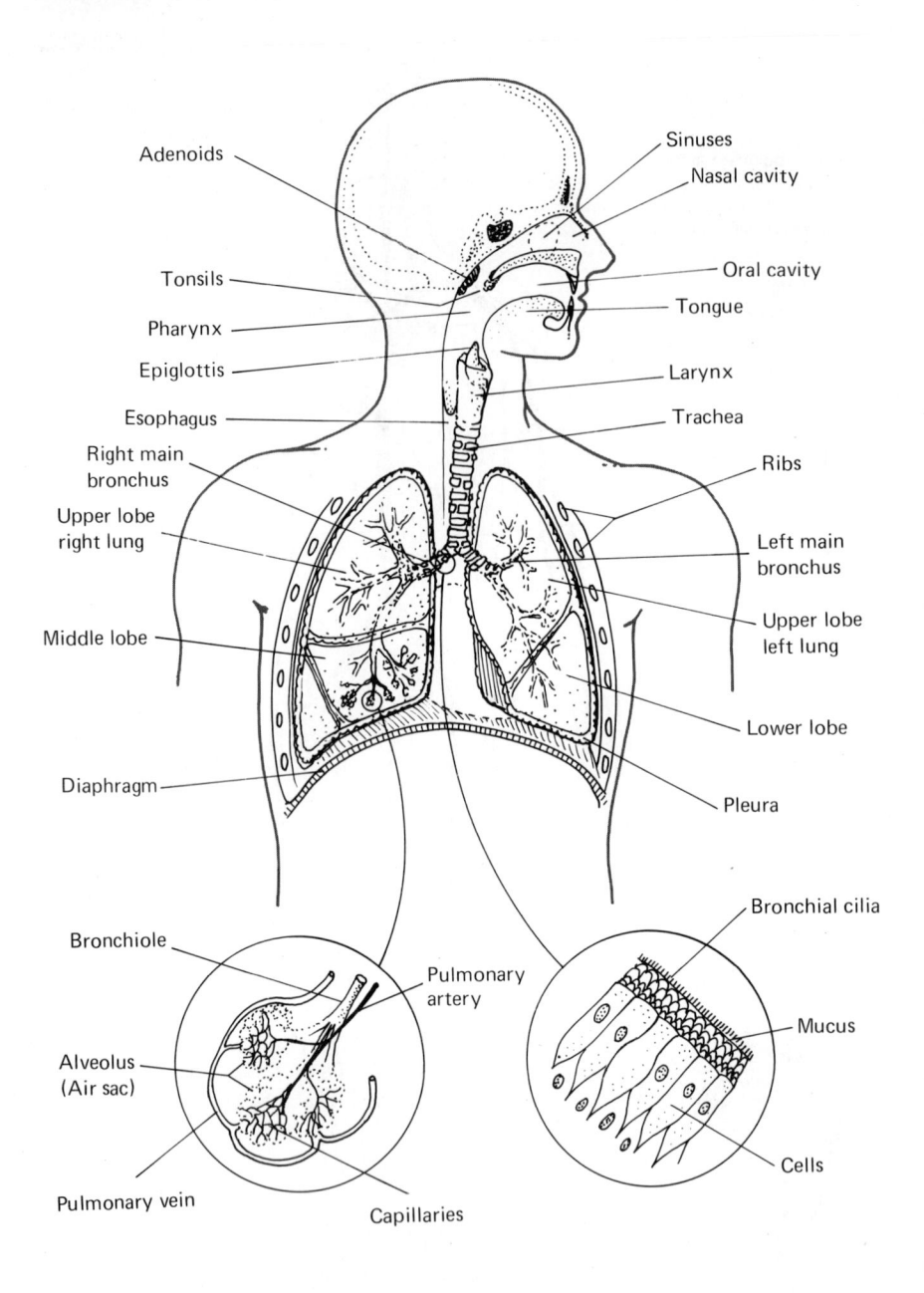

GLOSSARY

glossary

Abdomen Portion of the body between the chest and the pelvis, containing the stomach, intestines, and other organs.

Abortion Expulsion of the fetus before it is sufficiently developed to lead an independent existence outside of the uterus.

Absorption Passage of materials from the stomach and intestines into the circulatory system.

Acclimate To become accustomed to a new environment.

Acidosis General acid condition of the body.

Acute Severe but of short duration, as a disease or condition.

Afterbirth The placenta and fetal membranes expelled from the womb after childbirth.

Airway The breathing passage in the head or throat; or, a device used to keep the passageway open.

Allergen Any substance that produces an allergic reaction.

Allergy An abnormal sensitivity to a substance.

Alveoli Minute air sacs in the lungs through which respiratory exchanges take place.

Anaerobic Absence of oxygen.

Anaphylaxis An exaggerated type of sensitivity to a protein substance.

Aneurysm A ballooning or swelling of a blood vessel.

Angina pectoris A characteristic pain produced when oxygen supply to the heart muscle is inhibited.

[215]

Anoxia Diminished or inadequate oxygen supply in the blood and cells.

Antibiotic Any agent which kills or inhibits the growth of bacteria.

Antibody A substance produced within the body as a result of an infectious agent or allergy.

Anticoagulant A substance which prevents or inhibits the coagulation of blood.

Antidote Any substance used to combat the effects of a poison.

Antihistamine Any chemical compound which neutralizes or combats the physiologic effects of histamine, a chemical substance in the body which causes allergic reactions.

Antiseptic A substance or compound that inhibits or prevents the growth of micro-organisms.

Antitoxin A substance injected into the body to combat or neutralize the effect of poisonous substances secreted by various disease-producing bacteria.

Aorta The largest artery of the body.

Apoplexy Synonymous with stroke and cerebral vascular accident.

Appendectomy Removal of the appendix by surgery.

Appendicitis Inflammation of the appendix.

Arrest A stoppage of circulation or ventilation.

Arrhythmia Any abnormal rhythm of the heartbeat.

Arteriole A minute arterial branch.

Artery A vessel in which blood flows away from the heart, in the systemic circulation, carrying oxygenated blood.

Asphyxia Synonymous with anoxia; also termed suffocation.

Aspirate To breathe or suck (into the lungs).

Asthma An allergic condition characterized by wheezing and difficult breathing, especially when exhaling. Caused by constriction and spasms of the bronchial tubes.

Atherosclerosis Degeneration of the artery wall brought about by deposits and loss of elasticity, and causing reduction in size of the arterial opening.

Aura Premonition of impending seizure, commonly associated with epilepsy.

Auricles Upper chambers of the heart.

Autonomic nervous system The involuntary or sympathetic portion of the nervous system, over which there is no voluntary control.

Bacteria Rod-shaped micro-organisms, some of which are pathogenic (disease-producing).

Biological death Time at which irreversible damage occurs to the cells of the brain, usually four to six minutes following clinical death.

Block An obstruction in any part of the body, for example, blood vessel or intestine.

Bolus A mass of food ready to be swallowed, some of which may not be completely chewed.

Bradycardia A slow heart beat, usually between 40 and 60 beats per minute or slower.

Café coronary Death from an apparent heart attack, but actually brought on by food obstructing the trachea.

Capillary The smallest branch of an artery or vein.

Cardiac Referring to the heart.

Cardiac massage Rhythmic compression and relaxation of the heart performed on the outside of the body. The heart is squeezed between the sternum and the vertebrae.

Cardiovascular Referring to the circulatory system.

Carotid The two major arteries of the neck, supplying the head and brain with oxygenated blood. The carotid pulse is felt at the side of the neck, below the jaw.

Cartilage An elastic substance which covers the opposing surfaces of moving joints.

Caustic A corrosive chemical, alkaline in nature, which destroys tissue.

Cerebral vascular accident (CVA) Apoplexy or stroke.

Cervix The lower portion of the uterus, opening into the vagina.

Cesarean section Delivery of a baby by surgical incision into the uterus through the abdomen.

Chronic Lasting a long time or recurring often; said of a disease or condition.

Clinical death The moment when the heart stops beating and respiration ceases.

Coagulation time Time required for blood to clot.

Coma Unconsciousness.

Comatose The state of partial or complete unconsciousness.

Communicable dieases A contagious disease, one that can be transmitted from one person to another either directly by contact (via kissing, etc.) or indirectly (via sneezes, coughs, drinking glass, etc.).

Compress A clean or sterile pad or folded cloth used for applying pressure to a hemorrhaging wound.

Concussion A condition of the brain resulting from a violent blow or shock.

Congestion Stagnation of fluid in the tissues.

Constriction A narrowing or compression, especially of the pupils of the eye or of the blood vessels.

Contagious Used to describe a disease or condition which is readily transmitted by direct or indirect contact.

Contaminated That which is no longer clean or sterile; infected with microorganisms.

Glossary

Contraction Shortening of a muscle in action. In obstetrics, relates to the muscles opening the cervix prior to delivery of a baby.

Contusion A bruise.

Convulsion A series of involuntary muscular spasms; may affect the entire muscular system of the body or only a part.

CPR Cardiopulmonary resuscitation.

Cravat A special type of bandage made from a large triangular piece of cloth, usually muslin or cotton.

Crepitus The crackling sound or sensation produced by the grating of fractured bone ends.

Cricotracheostomy An incision into the trachea through the cricoid cartilage to obtain an airway in instances of respiratory obstruction.

Cryotherapy The therapeutic use of cold.

CVA Cerebral vascular accident, also known as stroke or apoplexy.

Cyanosis Blueness of the skin due to insufficient oxygenation.

Defecate To excrete feces, move the bowels.

Depressant Any agent which retards or slows a bodily function.

Dermis The layer of skin lying beneath the epidermis, or outermost layer.

Desensitization A process of making an individual less sensitive to allergens.

Diabetes Inability of the body to metabolize carbohydrates as a result of the failure of the pancreas to secrete enough insulin.

Diaphragm The large muscle between the chest cavity and the abdominal cavity; it plays a major role in breathing.

Diarrhea Abnormally frequent, liquidy bowel movement.

Dilation The process of expanding or enlarging, often associated with the pupils of the eye or blood vessels.

Disease Illness, sickness, abnormal state, interruption of body function.

Dislocation Out of normal position, usually referring to the position of the bones at a joint.

Edema Swelling caused by an abnormal amount of fluid in the tissues.

Electrocardiogram (ECG or EKG) A graph of the electrical pattern occurring during the contraction and relaxation of the heart muscle.

Electroencephalogram (EEG) A graph of the electrical impulses in the brain.

Embolus A transported blood clot or foreign matter which may cause a blockage in the circulatory system.

Emergency care The care, packaging, extrication, and transportation of an ill or injured individual by trained personnel until definitive treatment is begun or continued at a medical facility.

Emetic An agent which will induce vomiting.

Emphysema Infiltration of any tissue with air or gas, particularly within the lungs.

Epidermis The outermost layer of skin.

Epiglottis Cartilaginous lid of the larynx; when functioning properly it keeps food and foreign matter from entering the trachea.

Epilepsy A disorder of the central nervous system characterized by convulsions.

Esophagus The tube leading from the pharynx to the stomach.

Exsanguinate To hemorrhage so severely that all or most of the blood is expelled from the body.

Extricate To remove, as from a wrecked automobile or entrapment.

Fetus Unborn child.

Fibrillation Rapid twitching of a muscle due to independent action of its fibers; usually associated with the ventricles of the heart.

First aid The prompt, efficient care of an individual, whether injured or ill, until medical assistance becomes available.

Flail chest Injury in which three or more ribs are broken, each in two places. As a result, the segment of chest wall between the breaks collapses with each attempted breath, causing acute respiratory distress.

Fracture A break in the bone or the loss of continuity of the bone.

Frostbite Injury to the tissues as a result of exposure to cold.

Gangrene Local tissue death caused by constriction of its blood supply as a result of injury or illness.

Germ Any micro-organism, some being pathogenic (disease-producing) agents.

Groin Area of the body at the junction of the abdomen and the thigh.

Hallucination A disorder of perception; seeing or hearing things that are not there.

Heart block A short circuit in the electrical mechanism of the heart, causing the auricles and ventricles to beat independently.

Hematoma Blood clot; the collection of blood in the tissues as the result of injury or a broken blood vessel, usually just below the skin.

Hemoglobin The oxygen and carbon dioxide carrying mechanisms in red blood cells.

Hemophilia An inherited blood disease of males, passed through the female genes. Characterized by inability of the blood to clot.

Hemorrhage Bleeding.

Hemothorax Blood in the thoracic (chest) cavity.

Hyperglycemia An abnormally high amount of sugar in the blood.

Hyperinsulinism Too much insulin in the blood.

Hypersensitivity Increased or excessive sensitivity to a substance or stimulus.

Hypertension High blood pressure.

Hyperventilation Abnormally prolonged and deep breathing, altering the oxygen-carbon dioxide balance in the body.

Hypoglycemia Abnormally low level of sugar in the blood. The opposite of hyperglycemia.

Hypotension Low blood pressure.

Hysteria An emotional disturbance characterized by a lack of control over one's emotions.

Immobilization Holding firmly in place, as by a splint.

Infarction Death of tissue due to interference with the circulation to it. Often associated with the heart muscle.

Infection Invasion by living pathogenic micro-organisms of a part of the body where the conditions are favorable to their growth, and whence their toxins may gain access to and act injuriously upon the tissues.

Inflammation Condition characterized by pain, heat, redness, and swelling of tissues.

Ingestion Act of taking materials into the body by way of the mouth.

Insulin A hormone secreted by the pancreas, vital for metabolizing carbohydrates.

Intravenous (IV) Injection of medication or fluids directly into a vein, using a needle or tube system.

Intubation The act of inserting a tube into the larynx to relieve a respiratory obstruction.

Joint An area where bone ends meet, touch, or join.

Jugular vein The main blood vessel collecting the blood from the head and neck.

Laryngectomy Surgical removal of the larynx.

Larynx The voice box.

Lavage A washing out of the stomach, associated with ingested poisoning.

Ligament A tough band of fibrous tissue which connects bones about a joint.

Lockjaw Tetanus; a disease characterized by acute spasm of the jaw muscles which prevents the mouth from being opened.

Medulla oblongata Lowest part of the brain at the top of the spinal cord, housing the nerve centers of respiration, circulation, etc.

Metabolism The conversion of food into energy and waste products.

Miscarriage Synonymous with abortion; premature expulsion of the fetus.

Mucous membrane Thin tissue which lines many organs of the body and contains glands that secrete mucus.

Mucus A viscid, watery-like secretion which serves as a lubricant.

Myocardium The muscular structure of the heart.

Narcotic An addicting or habit-forming drug used to induce sleep or relieve pain.

Neurosis Emotional disorder characterized by anxiety, depression, phobias, and other reactions.

Occlusion Stoppage of a blood vessel due to a clot or embolus.

Palpable Feelable with one's hands.

Palpation The act of discerning normality or abnormality by feeling with the fingers.

Palpitation Abnormally rapid heartbeat.

Paralysis Stoppage of muscle function due to interference with its nerve supply.

Pathogenic Capable of producing a disease.

Peritoneum The sac which lines the inner wall of the abdominal cavity.

Peritonitis An inflammation or infection of the peritoneum.

Pharynx The passageway leading from the back of the mouth and nasal passages to the larynx.

Placenta Organ by which the unborn child is attached to the inside of the uterus and through which the child's body needs are supplied. Expelled after birth.

Plaque A hardened deposit on the walls of an artery. Causes artery to lose elasticity and may cause occlusion.

Plasma The fluid portion of the blood from which the red and white cells have been removed.

Pleura The glistening fibrous tissue sheath which lines the inner surface of the chest wall and envelops the lungs.

Pollen The male fertilizing element of a plant. May cause allergenic reaction in sensitive individuals.

Pneumonia An acute infection of the lungs.

Pneumothorax Air in the thoracic cavity.

Precordial thump A single sharp blow to the mid-portion of the sternum. It acts to reverse the heart's non-pumping action.

Premature birth Child born before the seventh month or weighing less than 5 to 5½ pounds at birth.

Prone Lying flat with the face downward.

Prostration Collapse.

Pulmonary edema An accumulation of fluid in the lungs.

Rabies A disease of the central nervous system affecting all warm-blooded animals. May be transmitted to humans by bite of affected animal.

Reflex Involuntary muscular action in response to a stimuli.

Regurgitation The spitting or vomiting up of the contents of the stomach.

Respiration The act of breathing, consisting of inspiration (inhaling) and expiration (exhaling). The process whereby living cells take in oxygen and give off carbon dioxide.

Resuscitation The act of reviving an unconscious individual by means of artificial ventilation with or without the use of cardiac massage.

Rigidity Extreme muscular tenseness.

Saline A solution of sodium chloride (salt) in water.

Skin graft A fragment of skin or other body tissue used for transplantation. Most often associated with burn therapy.

Spasm Strong involuntary contractions of a muscle or a set of muscles.

Sprain The stretching or partial tearing of the capsule or ligaments which surround a joint.

Sterilization The process of rendering any substance or material completely free of micro-organisms.

Stimulant Any agent that causes an increase in a normal or depressed bodily function.

Stoma An opening made in the trachea for purposes of breathing when the larynx has been surgically removed.

Strain An overstretching or tearing of a muscle or tendon.

Stroke A cerebral vascular accident; apoplexy.

Stupor State of partial or complete unconsciousness.

Subcutaneous Just beneath the skin.

Sunstroke A condition produced by extreme exposure to the sun or heat; also termed *heat stroke*.

Supine Lying flat on the back with the face up.

Suture Material such as catgut, thread, wire, etc., used for sewing or joining together the two edges of a wound.

Syncope Synonymous with fainting or psychogenic shock.

Tachycardia A very fast heart rate, usually between 100 to 160 beats per minute.

Tetanus Lockjaw; a disease characterized by convulsive action of the muscles.

Thorax That portion of the body between the neck and the abdomen.

Thrombus A clot which may occlude a blood vessel or a clot in one of the chambers of the heart.

Tissue Mass or group of cells of a particular type.

Toxemia A general poisoning of the body due to the spread of a local infection.

Toxic Poisonous.

Toxicity The degree of being poisonous.

Toxin Any poisonous substance formed by bacteria.

Toxoid A chemically modified toxin which when injected into the body stimulates the body to form protective substances against specific diseases.

Trachea Windpipe, respiratory passageway.

Tracheotomy Creation of an opening into the trachea by surgical incision through the neck to facilitate the passage of air or evacuation of secretions.

Trauma An injury, physical or emotional.

Umbilical cord Tough, elastic cord-like connection which attaches the fetus to the placenta and which must be cut after birth.

Unwitnessed arrest Situation in which a first aider finds an individual who is unconscious with no pulse and no breathing (*see* Witnessed arrest).

Uterus The womb; a hollow pear-shaped organ in which the fertilized ovum develops into a child.

Vaccine A substance introduced into the body to stimulate formation of antibodies in order to produce immunity to certain diseases.

Vagina Birth canal.

Vasoconstrictor Any drug which causes a constriction of the blood vessels and raises blood pressure.

Vasodilator Any nerve, drug, or agent which causes dilation of the blood vessels.

Vein A vessel in which blood flows toward the heart, in the systemic circulation, carrying carbon dioxide and waste products.

Ventilation The mechanical process of moving air into and out of the body.

Ventricles Lower chambers of the heart; the pumping chambers.

Venule A minute branch of a vein.

Virus An extremely small parasitic infectious micro-organism.

Vomitus Matter which is expelled from the body during the process of vomiting.

Witnessed arrest Situation in which a first aider is present with an individual as he goes into respiratory and circulatory arrest (*see* Unwitnessed arrest).

SELECTED BIBLIOGRAPHY

GENERAL FIRST AID CARE

AARON, JAMES E., A. FRANK BRIDGES, AND DALE O. RITZEL. *First Aid and Emergency Care, Prevention and Protection of Injuries.* New York: The Macmillan Company, 1972.

AMERICAN ACADEMY OF ORTHOPAEDIC SURGEONS. *Emergency Care of the Sick and Injured.* Chicago, Ill., 1971.

AMERICAN MEDICAL ASSOCIATION. *The Wonderful Human Machine.* Chicago, Ill., 1961.

AMERICAN NATIONAL RED CROSS. *Advanced First Aid and Emergency Care.* Garden City, N.Y.: Doubleday and Company, 1973.

──────. *Standard First Aid and Personal Safety.* Garden City, N.Y.: Doubleday and Company, 1973.

BRENNAN, WILLIAM T., AND DONALD J. LUDWIG. *Guide to Problems and Practices in First Aid and Civil Defense.* 2nd ed. Dubuque, Iowa: William C. Brown Company, 1970.

BYRD, OLIVER E., AND THOMAS R. BYRD. *Medical Readings on First Aid.* San Francisco: Boyd and Fraser Publishing Company, 1971.

CANADIAN RED CROSS SOCIETY, *Red Cross First Aid.* 3rd ed. Toronto, 1968.

COLE, WARREN H., AND CHARLES B. PRESTON. *First Aid Diagnosis and Management.* New York: Appleton-Century-Crofts, 1965.

CURRY, GEORGE J. *Immediate Care and Transportation of the Injured.* Springfield, Ill.: Charles C. Thomas Publishers, 1965.

ERVEN, LAWRENCE, W. *First Aid and Emergency Rescue.* Beverly Hills, Calif.: Glencoe Press, 1970.

Selected Bibliography

FLINT, THOMAS, JR., AND HARVEY D. CAIN. *Emergency Treatment and Management*. Philadelphia, Pa.: W. B. Saunders Company, 1970.

GARDNER, A. W., AND P. J. ROYLANCE. *New Essential First Aid*. London: Pan Books Ltd., 1967.

GOWING, DAN D., ed. *Ambulance Attendant Training Manual*. Philadelphia: Pennsylvania Department of Health, 1964.

GRANT, HARVEY, AND ROBERT MURRAY. *Emergency Care*. Bowie, Md.: Robert J. Brady Company, 1971.

HAFEN, BRENT Q., ALTON L. THYGERSON, AND RAY A. PETERSON, eds. *First Aid: Contemporary Practices and Principles*. Minneapolis, Minn.: Burgess Publishing Company, 1972.

HENDERSON, JOHN. *Emergency Medical Guide*. 4th ed. New York: McGraw-Hill Book Company, 1973.

IGEL, B. H. *First Aid*. Palo Alto, Calif.: Behavioral Research Laboratories, 1965.

KENNEDY, ROBERT H., ed. *Emergency Care of the Sick and Injured*. Philadelphia, Pa.: W. B. Saunders Company, 1966.

LEWIS, ARNOLD, ed. *Immediate Care of the Sick and Injured*. Sedgwick County, Kan.: Kansas Medical Society, 1966.

NATIONAL SAFETY COUNCIL. *Accident Facts*. Chicago, 1974.

OHIO TRADE AND INDUSTRIAL EDUCATION SERVICE, Division of Vocational Education. *Emergency Victim Care and Rescue*. 2nd ed. Columbus, Ohio: Department of Education, 1965.

RAFFERTY, MAX. *Emergency Care of the Sick and Injured*. Sacramento, California: State Department of Education, 1969.

ST. JOHN AMBULANCE ASSOCIATION. *First Aid*. 2nd ed. London: Hills and Lacy Ltd., 1965.

UNITED STATES ARMY. *Bandaging and Splinting*. Field Manual 8/50. Washington, D.C.: Government Printing Office, 1953.

———. *Transportation of the Sick and Wounded*. Field Manual 8/35. Washington, D.C.: Government Printing Office, 1966.

U.S. DEPARTMENT OF THE INTERIOR, BUREAU OF THE MINES. *First Aid*. Washington, D.C.: Government Printing Office, 1953.

———. *First Aid Instruction Course*. Washington, D.C.: Government Printing Office, 1970.

U.S. PUBLIC HEALTH SERVICE, OFFICE OF CIVIL DEFENSE. *Medical Self-Help Training Manual*. Washington, D.C.: Government Printing Office, 1965.

UNITED STATES NAVY. *Standard First Aid Training Course*. Navpers 100801-A. Washington, D.C.: Government Printing Office, 1955.

YOUNG, CARL B. *First Aid for Emergency Crews*. Springfield, Ill.: Charles C. Thomas Publishers, 1965.

———. *Transportation of the Injured*. Springfield, Ill.: Charles C. Thomas Publishers, 1958.

EMERGENCY MEDICAL SERVICES

AMERICAN COLLEGE OF SURGEONS, COMMITTEE ON TRAUMA. "Essential Equipment for Ambulances." *Bulletin of the American College of Surgeons*, 55: 7–13, 1970.

―――. "Standards for Emergency Ambulance Services." *Bulletin of the American College of Surgeons*, 52: 131–132, 1967.

AMERICAN MEDICAL ASSOCIATION, COMMISSION ON EMERGENCY MEDICAL SERVICES. *Developing Emergency Medical Services: Guidelines for Community Councils*. Chicago, n.d.

CHAYET, NEIL L. *Legal Implications of Emergency Care*. New York: Appleton-Century-Crofts, 1969.

"The Crisis in Emergency Care." *Medical World News*, December 4, 1970.

FARRINGTON, J. D. "Community Training Program for Ambulance Attendants." *Bulletin of the American College of Surgeons*, 53: 178–179, 1968.

―――. "Death in a Ditch." *Bulletin of the American College of Surgeons*, 52: 121–130, 1967.

―――, AND OSCAR P. HAMPTON. "A Curriculum for Training Emergency Medical Technicians." *Bulletin of the American College of Surgeons*, 54: 273–276, 1969.

GOLD, S. Y., AND G. F. GOLD. "First Aid and Legal Liability." *Journal of Health, Physical Education, and Recreation*, January, 1963.

HALL, G. E. "When Death Occurs: Some Practical Aspects." *Journal of the American Medical Association*, September 19, 1966.

HAMPTON, OSCAR P. "A Systematic Approach to Emergency Medical Services." *Archives of Environmental Health*, August, 1970.

JENKINS, E. R. "Helicopter Evacuation of Highway Injuries," *General Practitioner*, December, 1968.

LONDON, P. S. "Helicopters in Civilian Medical Services," *Journal of Trauma*, October, 1970.

NATIONAL ACADEMY OF ENGINEERING. *Ambulance Design Criteria*. Washington, D.C.: Government Printing Office, 1970.

NATIONAL ACADEMY OF SCIENCES, DIVISION OF MEDICAL SCIENCES. *Medical Requirements for Ambulance Design and Equipment*. Washington, D.C., 1968.

―――. *Training of Ambulance Personnel and Others Responsible for Emergency Care of the Sick and Injured at the Scene and During Transport*. Washington, D.C., 1968.

―――. *Accidental Death and Disability: The Neglected Disease of Modern Society*. Washington, D.C., 1966.

NATIONAL EDUCATION ASSOCIATION, NATIONAL COMMISSION OF SAFETY EDUCATION. *Who Is Liable for Pupil Injuries?* Washington, D.C., 1963.

TURNER, H. S., AND H. V. ELLINGSON. "Use of the Helicopter as an Emergency

[230] Selected Bibliography

Vehicle in the Civilian Environment." *Aerospace Medicine*, February, 1970.

U.S. PUBLIC HEALTH SERVICES. *Compendium of State Statutes on the Regulation of Ambulance Services, Operation of Emergency Vehicles, and Good Samaritan Laws*. Washington, D.C.: Government Printing Office, 1969.

CARDIOPULMONARY RESUSCITATION

AMERICAN HEART ASSOCIATION. *Emergency Measures in Cardiopulmonary Resuscitation, Discussion Guide*. New York: 1965.

BARNES, THOMAS A., AND JACOB S. ISRAEL. *Respiratory Therapy*. Bowie, Md.: Robert J. Brady Company, 1971.

GORDON, ARCHER S., ed. *Cardiopulmonary Resuscitation: Conference Proceedings*. Washington, D.C.: National Academy of Sciences–National Research Council, 1967.

HAUGEN, R. K. "The Café Coronary." *Journal of the American Medical Association*, October 12, 1963.

HEIMLICH, HENRY. "Pop Goes the Café Coronary." *Emergency Medicine*, June, 1974.

INTERNATIONAL ASSOCIATION OF LARYNGECTOMEES. *First Aid for Laryngectomees*. New York: American Cancer Society, 1962.

JUDE, JAMES R. *Closed Chest Cardiac Resuscitation: Methods–Indications–Limitations*. New York: American Heart Association, 1966.

———, AND JAMES D. ELAM. *Fundamentals of Cardiopulmonary Resuscitation*. Philadelphia, Pa.: F. A. Davis Company, 1965.

KOUWENHOVEN, W. B., JAMES R. JUDE, AND G. GUY KNICKERBOCKER. "Heart Activation in Cardiac Arrest." *Modern Concepts of Cardiovascular Disease*, February, 1961.

———. "Closed Chest Cardiac Massage." *Journal of the American Medical Association*, July 9, 1960.

NATIONAL ACADEMY OF SCIENCES, DIVISION OF MEDICAL SCIENCES. "Cardiopulmonary Resuscitation." *Journal of the American Medical Association*, October 24, 1966.

NATIONAL ACADEMY OF SCIENCES–NATIONAL RESEARCH COUNCIL AND AMERICAN HEART ASSOCIATION. "Standards for Cardiopulmonary Resuscitation and Emergency Cardiac Care." *Supplement to the Journal of the American Medical Association*, February 18, 1974.

SAFAR, PETER. ed. *Cardiopulmonary Resuscitation: A Manual for Physicians and Paramedical Instructors*. Bronxville, N.Y.: World Federation of Societies of Anesthesiologists, 1968.

STRINGER, LLEWELLYN W. *Emergency Treatment of Acute Respiratory Diseases*. Bowie, Md.: Robert J. Brady Company, 1973.

SOFT TISSUE INJURIES: BITES, BURNS

ARNOLD, R. E. *What to Do About Bites and Stings of Venomous Animals*. New York: The Macmillan Company, 1973.

Selected Bibliography [231]

ARTZ, C. P., AND E. REISS. *The Treatment of Burns.* Philadelphia, Pa.: W. B. Saunders Company, 1957.

COMMITTEE ON TRAUMA. "Guide to Initial Therapy of Burns." *Bulletin of the American College of Surgeons,* 52: 196–198, 1967.

CONANT, ROGER. *A Field Guide to the Reptiles and Amphibians.* New York: Houghton-Mifflin, 1958.

KLAUBER, LAURENCE M. *Rattlesnakes, Their Habits, Life-Histories, and Influence on Mankind.* 2nd ed. Berkeley, Ca.: University of California Press, 1972.

MCLAUGHLIN, HARRISON L. *Trauma.* Philadelphia, Pa.: W. B. Saunders Company, 1959.

MURRAY, R. "Electric Shock." *New England Journal of Medicine,* May 16, 1963.

NATIONAL ACADEMY OF SCIENCES–NATIONAL RESEARCH COUNCIL. "Statement on First Aid Therapy and on Hospital Care for Bites of Venomous Snakes." *Toxicon,* 1: 81–87, 1963.

NATIONAL SAFETY COUNCIL. "Shock: The Killer Hardly Anyone Knows." *Family Safety,* Summer, 1965.

———. "Tetanus, What Your Family Should Know About It." *Family Safety,* Summer, 1966.

———. "The Bashful Brown Spider." *School Safety,* March–April, 1969.

STARZL, T. E. "Treatment of Frostbite Today." *Consultant,* January, 1967.

STEBBINS, R. C. *A Field Guide to Western Reptiles and Amphibians.* New York: Houghton-Mifflin, 1966.

SKELETAL SYSTEM INJURIES

COMMITTEE ON TRAUMA. *The Measurement of Fractures and Soft Tissue Injuries.* 2nd ed. Philadelphia, Pa.: W. B. Saunders Company, 1965.

FARRINGTON, J. D. "Extrication of Victim–Surgical Principles." *Journal of Trauma,* 8: 493–512, 1968.

KOSSUTH, L. C. "Aquatic Rescue of Injured Personnel." *Journal of the Alabama Medical Association,* 35: 748–755, 1966.

———. "Immediate Care to Vehicle Accident Victims." *Postgraduate Medicine,* 41: 407–413, 1967.

———. "The Initial Movement of the Injured." *Military Medicine,* 132: 18–21, 1967.

———. "The Removal of Injured Personnel from Wrecked Vehicles," *Journal of Trauma,* 5: 703–708, 1965.

———. "Vehicle Accidents: Immediate Care to Back Injuries." *Journal of Trauma,* 6: 582–591, 1966.

POISONS AND POISONING

DASH, G. M. *Food Poisoning.* Chicago, Ill.: University of Chicago Press, 1965.

DREISBACH, ROBERT H. *Handbook on Poisoning.* 5th ed. Los Altos, Calif.: Lange Medical Publications, 1966.

[232] Selected Bibliography

MERCK AND COMPANY. *The Index of Chemicals and Drugs.* 7th ed. Rahway, N.J., 1960.

NATIONAL INSTITUTE OF ALLERGY AND INFECTIOUS DISEASES. *Poison Ivy, Oak, and Sumac.* Washington, D.C.: Government Printing Office, 1967.

NATIONAL CLEARINGHOUSE FOR POISON CONTROL CENTERS. *Bulletin*: May-June, 1974. Washington, D.C.: Government Printing Office.

U.S. DEPARTMENT OF AGRICULTURE. *Poison Ivy, Poison Oak, Poison Sumac.* Washington, D.C.: Government Printing Office, 1967.

VERHULTZ, HENRY L., AND JOHN CROTTY. "Poison Control Activities in the United States." *Journal of School Health*, February, 1967.

MEDICAL EMERGENCIES

AMERICAN HEART ASSOCIATION. *Facts About Heart and Blood Vessel Disease.* New York, 1966.

CONKLIN, GROFF. *Diabetes Unknown.* New York: Public Affairs Committee, 1963.

EPILEPSY FOUNDATION. *Answers to Some of the Most Frequently Asked Questions About Epilepsy.* Washington, D.C., n.d.

———. *Epilepsy: Its Causes and Treatment.* Washington, D.C., n.d.

GORDON, JOHN E., ed. *Control of Communicable Diseases in Man.* New York: American Public Health Association, 1970.

HUSZAI, ROBERT J. *Emergency Cardiac Care.* Bowie, Md.: Robert J. Brady Company, 1974.

JOHNS, E. B., W. C. SUTTON, AND L. WEBSTER. *Health for Effective Living.* 4th ed. New York: McGraw-Hill Book Company, 1966.

MELTZER, LAWRENCE E., ROSE PINNEO, AND J. RODERICK KITCHELL. *Intensive Coronary Care: A Manual for Nurses.* Bowie, Md.: The Charles Press Publishers, Inc., 1970.

NATIONAL INSTITUTES OF HEALTH, INSTITUTE OF NEUROLOGICAL DISEASES AND BLINDNESS. *Epilepsy, Hope Through Research.* Washington, D.C.: Government Printing Office, 1962.

———. *Epilepsy, Research Profile No. 10.* Washington, D.C.: Government Printing Office, 1965.

ORR, R. "Mobile Coronary Care." *New England Journal of Medicine*, January 15, 1970.

PANTRIDGE, J. F. AND A. A. ADGEY. "Pre-Hospital Coronary Care." *American Journal of Cardiology*, November, 1969.

STINSON, P. M., AND H. L. HODES. *A Manual for the Common Contagious Diseases.* 5th ed. Philadelphia, Pa.: Lea & Fiebger, 1956.

U.S. PUBLIC HEALTH SERVICE, DIVISION OF CHRONIC DISEASES. *Diabetes.* Washington, D.C.: Government Printing Office, n.d.

WHITE, GREGORY, J. *Emergency Childbirth, A Manual.* Franklin Park, Ill.: Police Training Foundation, 1958.

PSYCHOLOGICAL EMERGENCIES: ALCOHOL, DRUGS, DISTRESS

AMERICAN PSYCHIATRIC ASSOCIATION, *First Aid for Psychological Reactions in Disasters*, Washington, D.C., 1964.

BECK, AARON T., HARVEY RESNIK, AND DAN J. LETTIERI. *The Prediction of Suicide*. Bowie, Md.: The Charles Press Publishers, Inc., 1974.

BRECHER, EDWARD M., AND THE EDITORS OF CONSUMER REPORTS. *Licit and Illicit Drugs*. Boston, Mass.: Little, Brown, and Company, 1972.

FORNEY, ROBERT B., AND FRANCIS W. HUGHES. *Combined Effects of Alcohol and Other Drugs*. Springfield, Ill.: Charles C. Thomas Publishers, 1968.

GILLESPIE, DARWIN K. "Psychological First Aid." *Journal of School Health*, November, 1963.

GIRDANO, DOROTHY D., AND DANIEL A. GIRDANO. *Drugs—A Factual Account*. Reading, Mass.: Addison-Wesley Publishing Company, 1973.

INDIANA DEPARTMENT OF POLICE ADMINISTRATION. "Alcohol and Accidents." *The Role of the Drinking Driver in Traffic Accidents*. Bloomington, Ind.: Indiana University, 1963.

KATZ, BARNEY. *Understanding People in Distress*. New York: The Ronald Press, 1955.

KEATON, WILLIAM L. "Understanding Alcoholism." *Michigan Alcohol Education Journal*, January, 1966.

MACDONALD, J. M. "Suicide and Homicide by Automobile." *American Journal of Psychiatry*, 121: 366–370, 1964.

MATTHEWS, ROBERT A., AND LLOYD W. ROWLAND. *How to Recognize and Handle Abnormal People*. New York: The National Association for Mental Health, Inc., 1965.

MCGONAGLES, L. C. "Psychological Aspects of Disaster." *American Journal of Public Health*, April, 1964.

NATIONAL INSTITUTE ON ALCOHOL ABUSE AND ALCOHOLISM. *Facts About Alcohol and Alcoholism*. Washington, D.C.: Government Printing Office, 1974.

NORTHWESTERN UNIVERSITY TRAFFIC INSTITUTE. *Driving Under the Influence of Alcohol or Drugs*. Evanston, Ill.: Northwestern University Press, 1966.

RESNIK, HARVEY, AND HARVEY RUBEN, eds. *Emergency Psychiatric Care, The Management of Mental Health Crisis*. Bowie, Md.: The Charles Press Publishers, Inc., 1974.

U.S. DEPARTMENT OF HEALTH, EDUCATION, AND WELFARE. *Alcohol and Health: Special Report to the United States Congress*. Washington, D.C.: Government Printing Office, 1971.

INDEX

A

Abdominal pain, 150
Abdominal wounds, 66
Abortion, 176–77
Abrasions, 58
Acidosis, 141–42
Acid poisoning, 122–23
Airway blockage, 17, 19–21
　avoidance in breech delivery, 174–75
　Café coronary, 28–31
　clearing devices, 22–24
Alcohol abuse, symptoms, 158 (chart)
Alcohol blood levels, 154–55 (chart)
Alcohol reaction:
　delirium tremens, 156
　intoxication, 154–56
Alkali poisoning, 122–23
Allergic reactions (*see* Anaphylactic shock)
American Academy of Pediatrics, 119
American College of Surgeons, 9, 11
American Psychiatric Association, 151
Amputation, 53, 59, 60
Anaphylactic shock:
　care for, 82–83
　causing airway blockage, 17

Angina pectoris, 146
Anoxia, defined, 16
Antidotes for poisons, 124, 129 (chart)
Apoplexy, 148–49
Appendicitis, 150
Arm or leg presentation, in childbirth, 171–72
Arterial bleeding, 46–47
Artificial ventilation:
　of children and infants, 24
　effectiveness indicators, 28
　history, 15
　of newborn, 168–69
　procedures, 19–28
　rate, 24
Aspirin poisoning, 125, 128
Aura, 144
Avulsions, 60

B

Back fracture (*see* Spinal fracture)
Bag-mask resuscitation, 26
Bag of waters, 163
Bandages:
　cravat, 179–80, 186 (fig. 12.8)
　figure-of-eight, 182, 183 (fig. 12.4)

[235]

Bandages (*cont.*)
  head, 185–87 (fig. 12.9, 12.10)
  jaw, 187 (fig. 12.12)
  recurrent finger, 183, 185 (fig. 12.5)
  recurrent head, 183, 184 (fig. 12.6)
  roller gauze, 179–81
  spiral turns, 181–82 (fig. 12.3)
  torso, 186–87 (fig. 12.10)
  triangular, 179–80, 185–86
Barbiturate poisoning, 124–25
Bedbugs, 70–71 (chart)
Bee sting, 70–71 (chart)
Biological death, 32–33
Birth, 166–68
Bites:
  animal, 75–76
  human, 75
  insect, 69, 70–71 (chart)
  snake, 72–75
Blanket drag (*see* One-man emergency transfer)
Blanket lift, 201–2 (fig. 12.30)
Bleeding (*see* Hemorrhage)
Blisters, 112
Blood circulation, 46
Blue unconsciousness, 139 (chart)
Botulism food poisoning, 127 (chart)
Brachial artery, 50–51
Breathing, cessation of (*see* Artificial ventilation)
Breech birth, 172–75
Bruise, 57
Burns, 108–14
  chemical, 114
  electrical, 113
  eye, 69, 113–14 (fig. 7.4)
  first degree, 110
  radiating effect, 111 (fig. 7.3)
  second degree, 111
  severity by Rule of Nines, 109 (fig. 7.1)
  sunburn, 114
  superheated air, 113
  third degree, 111

C

Café coronary, 28–31
Capillary bleeding, 46–47

Carbon monoxide poisoning, 129–30
Cardiac arrest, 33–34
  unwitnessed, 34–37
  witnessed, 42–43
Cardiac massage, 34–37
  children and infants, 37
  dangers of, 39, 41, 42
  effectiveness indicators, 39
  improper, 41 (fig. 2.29)
  initiating and terminating, 43
Cardiogenic shock, 82
Cardiovascular accident (CVA), 148–49
Carotid artery, 9, 33, 42, 50–51
Chair carry, 200 (fig. 12.29)
Chemical burns, 114
Chest pain, 146–47
Chickenpox, 135 (chart)
Chigger bites, 70–71 (chart)
Childbirth, 164–71
  care of newborn, 168–69
  cutting umbilical cord, 170–71
  delivery complications:
    arm or single leg presentation, 171–72
    breech presentation, 172–75
    miscarriage, 176–77
    multiple births, 175–76
    prolapsed cord, 175
Chlorine poisoning, 130
Choke-Saver device, 29, 31
Circulation, blood, 33, 46, 211 (diagram)
Clavicle splint, 190–91 (fig. 12.17)
Clinical death, 32–33
Closed fracture, 90
Cold exposure, 116–18
  wind-chill factor, 115 (chart)
Coma:
  diabetic, 140, 142
  unknown, 135
Comminuted fracture, 91
Communicable diseases, 135, 136–37 (chart)
Concussion, 97–98
Congestive heart failure, 148
Contagious diseases, 135, 136–37 (chart)
Contractions, childbirth, 164–65
Contusions, 57

Index [237]

Convulsions, 143
Coral snake, 73 (fig. 4.9)
Coronary heart disease, 145–46
Coronary insufficiency, 146
Corrosive poisons, 122–23
Cravat bandaging, 179–80, 185–87
Crowning, 167
Cuts, 60

D

Death, 32–33
Delirium tremens, 156
Delivery, childbirth:
   complications, 171–76
   stages, 164–71
Depressed fracture, 91
Diabetes:
   diabetic coma, 141–42
   insulin shock, 142–43
Diabetic coma, 141–42
Diphtheria, 135 (chart)
Direct pressure hemorrhage control, 48–49
Dislocations, 102
Drug overdose, 124–25
Drug reactions, 151, 157–59

E

Elbow splint, 191–92 (fig. 12.18)
Electrical burns, 114
Electrical contact, 86
Electrocardiogram (EKG), 33
Electroencephalograph (EEG), 144
Embedded object, 63–64
Emergency care, defined, 3
Emergency medical identification, 8
Emergency Medical Services, 1
Emergency medical system, 3 (fig. 1.1), 4
Emetics, 124
Emotional illness, 151–53
Emotional shock, 84, 151–53
Encephalitis, 135 (chart)
Epilepsy, 143–45
Evaluation of ill and injured, 5–9
Examination of ill and injured, 5–8

Exposure (*see* Cold Exposure; Heat cramps)
External heart compression (*see* Cardiac massage)
Extrication survey, 11 (chart)
Eye:
   burns, 69, 113–14 (fig. 7.4)
   injuries, foreign objects, 67–69

F

Fainting, 84–85
Femoral artery, 50–51
Femur splint, 192–93 (fig. 12.20)
Figure-of-eight bandage, 182, 183 (fig. 12.4)
Finger splint, 192 (fig. 12.19)
First aid:
   definition, 2
   priorities, 9, 12
First aider's responsibilities, 3–4, 12–14
First degree burn, 110
Fluids and shock care, 80, 82
Food poisoning, 126–28
Fractures:
   causes, 89–90
   classification, 90–91
   general procedures, 95–96
   indicators, 92–94, (fig. 6.4)
   lower jaw, 98–99
   pelvis, 96
   skull, 97
   spine, 99–101
   types, described, 91–92
Frostbite, 116–18
Full backboard splint, 195–96 (fig. 12.25)

G

German measles, 135 (chart)
Glue sniffing, 159 (chart)
Good Samaritan statutes, 13 (chart)
Grand mal seizure, 144
Greenstick fracture, 91
Gunshot wound, 64

H

Half backboard splint, 196–98, 197 (fig. 12.26)
Hallucinogens, 159 (chart)
Hammock carry, 203–4 (fig. 12.32)
Head bandaging, 183, 184 (fig. 12.6), 185, 186 (fig. 12.9), 187 (fig. 12.11)
Head injury, 97–98
Heart anatomy, 210 (diagram)
Heart disorder:
    angina, 146
    congestive heart failure, 148
    coronary heart disease, 145–46
    coronary insufficiency, 146
    myocardial infarction, 147–48
Heat cramps, 108
Heat exhaustion, 106–7
Heat stroke, 107–8
Heimlich maneuver, 29, 30 (fig. 2.7), 31
Hematoma, 57
Hemorrhage:
    amputation, 53
    classification, 46
    control methods:
        direct pressure, 48–49
        indirect pressure, 49–51
        tourniquet, 51–53
    external, 47–48
    internal, 54–55
    in miscarriage, 176–77
    nose bleeds, 53–54
Hip fracture, 96
Humerus splint, 190 (fig. 12.16)
Hyperimmune serum, 76
Hyperventilation, 31–32

I

Identification tags, 8
Impacted fracture, 91
Incisions, 60
Indirect pressure hemorrhage control, 49–51
Infant:
    artificial ventilation, 24
    care of newborn, 168–69

Infection, 61–62
Infectious hepatitis, 135 (fig. 9.1)
Influenza, 135 (chart)
Insect bites, 69, 70–71 (chart)
Insignias, emergency medical, 8
Insulin shock, 142–43
Internal hemorrhage, 54–55
Intoxication, 154–56, 158
Ipecac, syrup of, as emetic, 124

J

Jaw bandaging, 187 (fig. 12.12)
Jaw fracture, 98–99

K

Knee splint, 194 (fig. 12.23)
Knee-chest position:
    breech presentation, 172, 173 (fig. 11.12)
    prolapsed cord, 175 (fig. 11.15)

L

Labor pains, 164–65
Lacerations, 60
Laryngectomee:
    anatomy, 27 (fig. 2.14)
    medical identification, 8
    resuscitation, 27–28
Lead poisoning, 133–34
Legal liability, 13–14
Lifting techniques (*see* Transporting techniques)
Lockjaw, 62–63
Longitudinal fracture, 92
Lower jaw fracture, 98–99
Lower leg splint, 193 (fig. 12.21)

M

Marijuana, 159 (chart)
Measles, 135 (chart)
Medic Alert Foundation, 8

Medical identification, 8, 140, 142
Meningitis, 135 (chart)
Miscarriage, 176–77
Mononucleosis, 135 (chart)
Mosquito bite, 70–71 (chart)
Mouth-to airway resuscitation, 24–26
Mouth-to-mouth resuscitation, 21
Mouth-to-nose resuscitation, 24
Mouth-to-stoma, 27–28
Multiple births, 175–76
Multiple fracture, 92
Mumps, 136 (chart)
Mushroom poisoning, 126 (chart)
Myocardial infarction, 147–48

N

Narcotics, 158 (chart)
National Safety Council, 69
Neck fracture, 99–101
Neurogenic shock, 86
Nitroglycerine, 146
Nose bleed, 53–54

O

Oblique fracture, 92
One-man emergency transfer, 198–99 (fig. 12.27)
Open fracture, 91

P

Pasteur treatment, 76
Patella splint, 194 (fig. 12.23)
Pelvic splint, 193 (fig. 12.22)
Pelvis fracture, 96
Petit mal seizure, 144
Petroleum distillates, 123–24
Pit viper snakes, 73 (fig. 4.9)
Placenta, 164, 169–71
Pneumothorax, 64–66
Poison:
    antidotes, 129 (fig. 8.3)
    barbiturate, 124–25
    carbon monoxide, 129–30
    chlorine, 131
    corrosive, 122–23

Poison (*cont.*)
    entry routes, 121
    food, 126–28
    indicators, 121–22
    lead, 133–34
    noncorrosive, 124
    petroleum distillates, 123–24
    plants, contact, 132 (chart), 133
    salicylate, 125, 128
    tear gas, 131
Poison control centers, 119–21
Poison ivy, oak, sumac, 132 (chart), 133
Poliomyelitis, 136 (chart)
Precordial thump, 42
Pregnancy, 163–64
    accident during, 171
Premature birth, 163
Pressure dressing, 48–49
Pressure point (hemorrhage control), 49–51
Prolapsed cord, 175
Psychogenic shock, 84–85
Psychological first aid, 151–53
Pulse:
    absence of, 33–34, (fig. 2.19)
    as vital sign, 9
Puncture, 60
Pupils of eye:
    as indicator of cardiac arrest, 33, 34 (fig. 2.20)
    as vital signs, 9

R

Rabies, 75–76
Recurrent finger bandage, 183, 185 (fig. 12.5)
Recurrent head bandage, 183, 184 (fig. 12.6)
Red unconsciousness, 138 (chart)
Respiration:
    physiology, 16
    as vital sign, 9
Respiratory arrest, 18–19
Respiratory system, 212 (diagram)
Resuscitation (*see also* Artificial ventilation)
    bag-mask, 26

Index

Resuscitation (cont.)
  mouth-to-airway, 24–26
  mouth-to-mouth, 21
  mouth-to-nose, 24
  mouth-to-stoma, 27–28
  recovery rates, 16 (graph)
Resuscitube devices, 25
Rib splint, 194 (fig. 12.24)
Roller gauze bandaging, 179–80, 181–85
Rule of Nines, 109 (fig. 7.1)

S

Salicylate poisoning, 125, 128
Salmonella food poisoning, 127 (chart)
Scarlet fever, 136 (chart)
Scorpion bite, 70–71 (chart)
Second degree burn, 111
Sedatives, 158 (chart)
Seizures (see Epilepsy)
Serrated fracture, 92
Shellfish poisoning, 126 (chart)
Shock:
  anaphylactic, 17, 82–83
  cardiogenic, 82
  cyclic effects, 78 (fig. 5.1)
  electrical contact, 86
  emotional, 84
  neurogenic, 86
  psychogenic, 84–85
  traumatic, 77–82
Six-man lift and carry, 205–6 (fig. 12.33)
Skeletal system, 101, 209 (diagram)
Skull fracture, 97
Sleeping pills (see Barbiturate poisoning)
Sling, 189–90 (fig. 12.15)
Smallpox, 136 (chart)
Snake bites, 72–75
Spider bite, 70–71 (chart)
Spinal fracture, 99–101
Spinal splint:
  full backboard, 195–96 (fig. 12.25)
  half backboard, 196–98 (fig. 12.26)
Spiral fracture, 92
Spiral turn bandaging, 181–82 (fig. 12.3)

Splinting:
  clavicle, 190–91 (fig. 12.17)
  elbow, 191–92 (fig. 12.18)
  femur, 192–93 (fig. 12.20)
  finger, 192 (fig. 12.19)
  humerus, 190 (fig. 12.16)
  lower leg, 196 (fig. 12.21)
  patella, 194 (fig. 12.23)
  pelvis, 193 (fig. 12.22)
  rib, 194 (fig. 12.24)
  spine (see Spinal splint)
  wrist/forearm, 189–90 (fig. 12.15)
Splinting principles, 95
Splints:
  commercial, 188 (fig. 12.13)
  fixation, 189
  improvised, 189 (fig. 12.14)
  traction, 189
Sprains, 101
Staphylococcal food poisoning, 126 (chart)
Stimulants, 159 (chart)
Stoma, 27
Strain, 102–3
Strep throat, 136 (chart)
Stress fracture, 92
Stretcher carry, 206 (fig. 12.34)
Stroke, 148–49
Suicide, 157, 160–61
Sunburn, 114
Sunstroke, 107–8
Superheated air, 113
Swallowing the tongue, 17

T

Tarantula bite, 70–71 (chart)
Tear gas poisoning, 131
Tetanus, 62–63
Third degree burn, 111
Three-man hammock carry, 203–4 (fig. 12.32)
Three-man lift and carry, 202–3 (fig. 12.31)
Tick bite, 70–71 (chart)
Torso bandaging, 186–87 (fig. 12.10)
Tourniquet, 51–53
Traction splinting, 189

Tranquilizers, 158 (chart)
Transporting techniques:
 blanket lift, 201–2 (fig. 12.30)
 chair carry, 200 (fig. 12.29)
 one-man emergency transfer, 198–99 (fig. 12.27)
 six-man lift and carry, 205–6 (fig. 12.33)
 stretcher carry, 206 (fig. 12.34)
 three-man hammock carry, 203–4 (fig. 12.32)
 three-man lift and carry, 202–3 (fig. 12.31)
 two-man carry, 199 (fig. 12.28)
Transverse fracture, 92
Traumatic shock, 77–82
Triangular bandaging, 179–80, 185–87
Trichinosis, 127 (chart)
Tuberculosis, 136 (chart)
Two-man carry, 199 (fig. 12.28)
Typhoid fever, 136 (chart)

U

Umbilical cord, 167, 168, 170–71, 175
Unconsciousness, 135, 138–40
Unidote, 124
Universal antidote, 124

V

Venous bleeding, 46–47
Venous pooling, 78

Vertebra, 100 (fig. 6.5)
Vertebral fracture (*see* Spinal fracture)
Vital signs, 9–10 (fig. 1.4)

W

White unconsciousness, 138–39 (chart)
Whooping cough, 136 (chart)
Wind-chill factor, 115 (chart)
Wounds, 57–58, 60–61
 abrasion, 58
 amputation, 60
 animal bite, 75–76
 avulsion, 60
 crushing, 60
 embedded object, 63–64
 eye, 67–69
 genital organ, 67
 gunshot, 64
 human bite, 75
 insect bite, 69, 70–71 (chart)
 incision, 60
 laceration, 60
 open abdominal, 66
 open chest, 64–66
 puncture, 60
 snake bite, 72–75
Wrist/forearm splint, 189–90 (fig. 12.15)

X

Xiphoid process, 35 (fig. 2.22)